# HOMEOPATHIC REMEDIES FOR

# THE STAGES OF LIFE

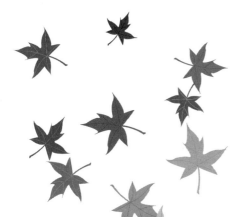

# HOMEOPATHIC REMEDIES

# FOR THE STAGES OF LIFE

## INFANCY, CHILDHOOD, AND BEYOND

## Didier Grandgeorge, M.D.
### Homeopathic Pediatrician

Translated from the original French
by Jennie Taylor

Foreword by Dana Ullman

**North Atlantic Books**
**Berkeley, California**

**Homeopathic Educational Services**
**Berkeley, California**

Published by

North Atlantic Books                    Homeopathic Educational Services
P.O. Box 12327                          2036 Blake Street
Berkeley, California 94712               Berkeley, California 94704

Cover and book design by Jennifer Dunn
Printed in the United States of America

*Homeopathic Remedies for the Stages of Life: Infancy, Childhood, and Beyond* is sponsored by the Society for the Study of Native Arts and Sciences, a non-profit educational corporation whose goals are to develop an educational and crosscultural perspective linking various scientific, social, and artistic fields; to nurture a holistic view of arts, sciences, humanities, and healing; and to publish and distribute literature on the relationship of mind, body, and nature.

---

North Atlantic Books are available through most bookstores. To contact North Atlantic directly, call 800-337-2665 or visit our website at www.northatlanticbooks.com.

Substantial discounts on bulk quantities of North Atlantic books are available to corporations, professional associations, and other organizations. For details and discount information, contact the special sales department at North Atlantic Books.

---

Library of Congress Cataloging-in-Publication Data

Grandgeorge, Didier.
    [Homéopathie chemin de vie. English]
    Homeopathic remedies for the stages of life : infancy, childhood,
and beyond / by Didier Grandgeorge ; translated from the original French
by Jennie Taylor.
        p. cm.
Includes index.
ISBN 1-55643-409-X (pbk.)
    1. Homeopathy. I. Title

RX71 .G7613 2002
615.5'32—dc21
                                                              2001056261

            1  2  3  4  5  6  /  06  05  04  03  02

# ACKNOWLEDGMENTS

Many thanks to my family, who patiently put up with my constant absences during the writing of this book, and especially to my wife Catherine and my children Yan, Bastien, and Pauline.

I would also like to thank Martine and Jean-Pierre Bourbon for their help. Without them, this book could never have been written.

The homeopathic physician does well when he trots the little
Johnnies and the little Susies on his knee and takes a good,
fair observation of their ability and of what they lack,
and understands how to build up what is lacking. Is not that
in itself worth working for?

J.T. Kent
*Lectures of Homeopathic Materia Medica*

# TABLE OF CONTENTS

# FOREWORD

Homeopathy has its own funny language. In *Homeopathic Remedies for the Stages of Life*, Dr. Didier Grandgeorge uses homeopathic language and terminology that may be unfamiliar to some readers and therefore requires a little explanation. An example of this language is the convention Grandgeorge employs by using a homeopathic medicine or remedy to refer to a type of person. I will endeavor here to explain this convention by introducing the reader to some basic homeopathic concepts and practices.

Instead of diagnosing a person as having a specific disease, as is done in conventional medicine, homeopaths usually define the disease the person has based on the medicine that is being prescribed for the sick person. Although this may at first seem a little strange, there is a profound logic to it.

A person is not simply a "kidney disease," a "colitis," a "fibroid," or a "cancer." A person is the totality of his or her physical and psychological characteristics and symptoms, and this totality is a dynamic, evolving system. The fact that conventional medicine reduces a person and his/her totality into a specific, limited, and usually localized pathology is quite strange in its own right.

In comparison, homeopaths understand that all diseases are part of a larger *syndrome*, that is, the whole body is influenced by infection and stress, and the whole body is aroused in its efforts to defend and heal itself from this perturbation. The human body is an incredibly complex web of small systems that are interconnected, and when one part of the web is affected, the entire web feels it, even if only minimally.

What is also important in understanding homeopathy is that symptoms are not usually evidence of the body's breakdown but instead are generally evidence of the body's defensive reaction and effort to defend and heal itself. This perspective—that symptoms are an integral part of the body's immune and defense system—is a modern understanding of stress theory and pathology.

Anyone who has ever been to a professional homeopath knows that homeopaths conduct an incredibly detailed interview, uncovering a wide variety of common, uncommon, and sometimes strange and unique symptoms in a person, and then ultimately prescribe a homeopathic medicine for that person and his/her own syndrome of physical and psychological symptoms.

To say that a person has a migraine headache or a peptic ulcer or an anxiety disorder simply does not do justice to the complexity of the various features of the person and the dis-ease he or she is experiencing. Instead, homeopaths describe the disease that the person has by saying, for example, that Joe Smith has an "Arsenicum album" disease *(Arsenicum album* is the Latin name for a common homeopathic medicine, arsenic. Homeopathic medicines are referred to by their Latin names because homeopaths want and need to be as precise as possible in describing the plant, mineral, or animal species that is the source of the medicine.).

Calling the disease by the name of the medicine gives the homeopath and fellow homeopaths (as well as educated consumers) a better, more detailed description of the complex syndrome of symptoms that the person is experiencing.

At first blush, calling someone a "Mercurius" person may sound strange, but if you know something about this medicine, this name provides a considerably more rich and sophisticated body of information than to say that this person has a peptic ulcer.


## APPRECIATING AND USING THIS BOOK

This book describes many homeopathic medicines and the syndrome of symptoms that each represents. What is unique about this book is that it is one of the first to describe the medicines in the light of developmental stages of a person's life. Understanding normal developmental stages is actually quite important in selecting a medicine for a person because a homeopath generally places more emphasis on a person's symptom if that symptom is unusual or unique. Such unusual or unique symptoms help the homeopath select a medicine that is more individualized to the sick person.

This book will help guide you to homeopathic medicines that are commonly indicated for dealing with the specific developmental problems that emerge at different stages in a person's life. Please keep in mind that we all go through life at our own pace, and that various events, experiences, and illnesses can speed up or slow down advancement to the next stage, and even reverse or revert one to an earlier stage. Because of this, don't read the information in each chapter as useful only for people in a specific age group. Each chapter can provide instructive and useful information about homeopathic medicines to people at any age in their lives.

Now that you've learned something about how to speak "homeopathic," you may want to begin teaching others the wisdom of this language. Although those of us who speak homeopathic are presently in a minority, this is changing very rapidly. And in any case, this language simply makes sense.

**Dana Ullman, MPH**

Author of *Everybody's Guide to Homeopathic Medicines* (with Stephen Cummings, MD), *Homeopathy A-Z, Essential Homeopathy, The Consumer's Guide to Homeopathy,* and *Homeopathic Medicines for Children and Infants*

# PREFACE TO
# THE AMERICAN EDITION

Here it is at last, the English version of *Homeopathie, chemin de vie*, thanks to Jennie Taylor's passionate work and Dana Ullman's helpful supervision. The book demonstrates a philosophic view of life as seen through the prism of homeopathic medicine. The human journey is described through all of its successive stages, from the initial selfish love to the final altruistic love. The human body and its various sicknesses, whether acquired or hereditary, are nothing more than the result of the struggle that the spirit faces along its path towards the Light, the Knowledge. Trapped within the matter that gives it motion, this spirit is the prey of the internal predators that push it to regress to the early selfish stages of development. But the spirit defeats its aggressors in the struggle that reveals the honor of mankind.

Does this bring us closer to the Truth, the White Light, or to Love in its three dimensions? Here the author presents a path that is worthy of diving into with all your energy! Homeopathic medicine's advantage, thanks to the dynamic remedies it proposes, is that it gives us the strength to overcome the obstacles that stand in our way. The symbolism of the human body is the symbolism of words, which serve as a precise tool, allowing us to understand and move forward.

My dear friends and readers, my best wishes are with you as you embark upon the enlightened path offered within!

**Didier Grandgeorge**
Marseille, July 6, 2001

# INTRODUCTION

After many years spent at the bedsides of my young patients, trying to find the source of their problems and help them through their illnesses, a number of ideas and theories started to formulate in my mind which I felt the need to put down in writing.

My medical career really began at the age of sixteen, when I broke my leg and was introduced to the world of hospitals. This experience led to a break in family tradition—we were expected to study mathematics and become engineers, and that was all. Nevertheless, I went on to study medicine and discovered an entire Art hidden behind my chosen discipline, despite the desire of some in our Western world to claim medicine as a purely scientific domain.

Personal health problems, in the form of allergies, finally led me to discover homeopathy—a form of treatment that was ignored or even denigrated by my superiors. And yet it was the only thing that had ever given me relief!

A subsequent interest in psychiatry and psychoanalysis showed me that everything experienced in childhood is stored and repressed into the depths of our unconscious.

It was while training to become a hospital intern that I took my first steps in professional practice. As an armed services volunteer, I managed to secure a post in Gabon, at the heart of the West African jungle. My desire to go to Africa was motivated by an interest in the developing world, an admiration for Dr. Albert Schweitzer, and perhaps also a yearning for adventure in the style of *Tintin in the Congo*. At that time, Africa represented for me the childhood of humanity.

After many obstacles and diversions, I finally arrived in Mimongo, land of the Mitzogo tribe. They greeted me with the words: "Your name is N'ganga Missoko—'He Who Heals All.'

You have returned to us and you will leave again." My purpose was to introduce these people, who had no written language of their own, to the richness and efficacy of modern medicine. In return, they taught me another kind of medicine—one that proved particularly effective for treating mental illnesses and for healing the rifts between body and soul. These people lived in a world of ever-changing spirits, and my experiences with their Witchdoctors, who served as both priests and physicians, revealed to me a new and exciting dimension.

On my return to France, I decided to specialize in pediatrics and continued my studies at Grenoble in the foothills of the French Alps. But a page had been turned and, no longer satisfied with modern techniques and treatments, I became one of the first students at Dr. Robert Bourgarit's newly established School of Homeopathy. Homeopathy fulfilled all my expectations, thanks to its ability to bridge the gap between psychoanalysis and "organic" medicine— areas that seemed irrevocably separated in modern medicine.

I found that children reacted particularly well to these tiny doses. The efficacy of homeopathic medicine was proved consistently by my own children and then confirmed by the hospital patients I cared for during many a night duty. But very few of my colleagues, who were also witness to these cures, chose to enter a field that demands so much personal investment.

Subsequently, I set myself up as a Homeopathic Pediatrician in the Côte d'Azur, where I was warmly received by the locals. This was partly thanks to the renown of the former homeopathy clinic at Saint Raphael (near Cannes), established by a certain Dr. Chargé at the end of the nineteenth century. Dr. Chargé succeeded in bringing together the expertise and knowledge of homeopathic doctors from all over France in his Ecole Hahnemannienne (Hahnemannian School). I and the other members of this Ecole still meet once every fortnight, in order to study the *Materia Medica* in greater depth and unearth its many hidden treasures. Our aim is to identify the thread which runs through each remedy and links its many thousands of symptoms, and the results of our work now extend to several volumes (published in France under the title *L'Homéopathie Exactement*).

It was with this same objective in mind that I published my own book *The Spirit of Homeopathic Medicines: Essential Insights to 300 Remedies* (North Atlantic Books, 1998). I wished to share our group's knowledge and insights with a wider audience, and the fact that this book has already been translated from the original French into Russian, Romanian, Italian, Spanish, English and German shows how well it has been received.

I have given you a brief summary of my life because this book is the result of all my experiences. It looks at the symbolism of human life and development, from conception through to death, and illustrates each successive stage with those homeopathic remedies which best characterize it.

Also used throughout are examples of Kabalistic phonetics—a Hebrew esoteric science that teaches us that every word of a language may contain numerous hidden meanings and connotations. The Israelites recognized this and applied it to every word, except for that which was never to be pronounced—the name of God or *yod hev vav hev*.

What we need to realize is that the human brain works along the same lines as Kabalistic phonetics. As homeopaths, understanding this enables us to decipher the unconscious messages hidden in the words of our patients and the names of our remedies.

Ultimately, the subject of this book is life itself, as the ultimate path of initiation. I invite you to accompany me along this path, as it leads us through the three dimensions of love.

**Didier Grandgeorge**
8 December 1997

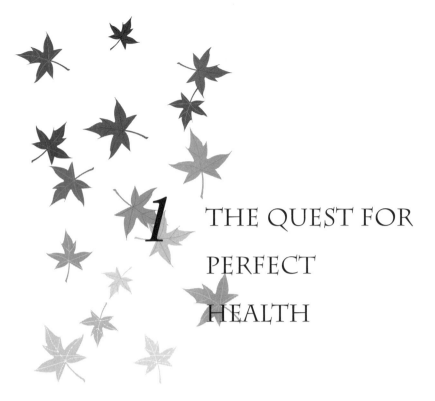

# 1    THE QUEST FOR PERFECT HEALTH

Christian Samuel Hahnemann, the brilliant nineteenth century founder of modern homeopathy, requested the following epitaph to be inscribed on his tomb:

*There are two treasures in life—perfect health and a clear conscience. Homeopathy provides the first; the second is acquired through love of God and our fellow man.*

What exactly is "perfect health?" According to the dictionary, health is the state of being "bodily and mentally vigorous and free from disease." In our modern, materialistic world, diseases are often thought to be caused by external agents such as bacteria and viruses, or else by wearing out of the organism, exposure to various pollutants, and human weakness for substances such as alcohol and tobacco. It is often assumed, for instance, that a sore throat will lead to bacterial infection of the tonsils and should therefore be treated with a course of antibiotics, in order to destroy the "invaders."

However, just like the nine-headed Hydra of Greek mythology, which grew two new heads in place of every one that was cut off, diseases often recur—leading to repeated doses of antibiotics and a consequent deterioration in health. Chronic illness sets in and the patient become dependent on ever more toxic drugs.

It can be argued that certain vaccines have wiped out previously unavoidable childhood illnesses. But in their place, more and more children and adults now suffer from allergies for which allopathic medicine offers no real solution. Asthmatics, for example, become slaves to their inhalers and daily doses of steroids, which they then find very difficult to stop. How is it that doctors, who every day are exposed to the bacteria and viruses of their suffering patients, don't become infected and fall ill more often? Could it be that these infective agents are blessed with intelligence and consciously decide to spare the healthcare workers? Of course not!

It doesn't take much to realize that, while bacteria and viruses are certainly contributory factors in disease, they are not in themselves enough to *cause* disease. First and foremost, the affected organism must have been unable to resist these intruders. A healthy immune system puts up an effective resistance and thereby protects us from disease. It is only when the basic soil of the organism is inadequate that illness sets in.


## THE SOIL OF DISEASE

Another way of approaching diseases is to look at the "soil" they grow from—in other words, the energetic state of the patient.

In his *Organon of Medicine* (Boericke, Sixth Edition), Hahnemann tells us that "In the healthy condition of man, the spiritual vital force (autocracy), the dynamis that animates the material body (organism), rules with unbounded sway, and retains all the parts of the organism in admirable, harmonious, vital operation, as regards both sensations and functions, so that our indwelling, reason-gifted mind can freely employ this living, healthy instrument for the higher purposes of our existence."

In spite of our materialistic Western culture, we all have a sense of this vital force inside us. Returning from a good holiday, we talk of having "recharged our batteries"—meaning that we're in good shape and feel rejuvenated. Conversely, we're only too aware of how certain situations can cause a drop in our energy, leaving us feeling "drained" and overcome with negativity.

Another Greek Myth—the Barrel of the Danaids—serves as a striking metaphor for these energy drains. The Danaids were the fifty daughters of Danaus, the King of Argos, who were forced to marry the fifty sons of Aegyptus. Because they had been married against their will, all but one of the Danaids stabbed their husbands to death on their wedding night. As punishment for their crimes, they were condemned to spend eternity in the Underworld, ladling water into a barrel full of holes.

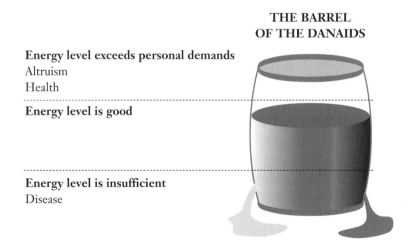

**THE BARREL
OF THE DANAIDS**

**Energy level exceeds personal demands**
Altruism
Health

**Energy level is good**

**Energy level is insufficient**
Disease

The barrel of this myth represents the human body, while the water represents energy. We are constantly drawing energy from the sun, food, and air, as well as from the love given out by others. But we are also constantly losing this energy through our own holes, of which we are mainly unaware.

A good state of health means that, despite the holes, we are receiving enough energy to keep our internal resources at an adequate level and resist any assault on our health. However, if there are too many holes or the holes are too large, the level inside the barrel falls. We are no longer able to resist external influences and disease takes a hold.

One way to slow down the disease's progress is to increase the energy supply, but if the holes are still there then the disease merely becomes chronic. It is only by plugging the holes in the barrel that we can hope to restore order, since this allows our energy levels to rise again—back up to, and even beyond, those required for good health. Every homeopath knows that when a patient has truly recovered, s/he experiences a new lease of life. In some cases, the barrel can even start to overflow with energy. The person finds they have enough not only for themselves but for others as well, and they are able to use some of these additional resources to accomplish great acts of altruism.

But how to find and plug the holes in people's barrels? According to the myth, the Danaids' destruction of their husbands and marriages symbolizes our own failure to go inside and unite the various aspects of ourselves. We need to dive into our own Unconscious, in order to confront our Shadow and inner beasts.

The conscious mind is just the tip of a very large iceberg. The vast majority of this huge block of ice lies hidden, and manipulates us without our knowledge. According to the Bible, having created man, God gave him dominion over all the animals and brought each one to him for naming—"and whatsoever Adam called every living creature, that was the name thereof." This doesn't mean that Adam literally went around identifying the lion, the giraffe, the elephant etc, but that it is the responsibility of each

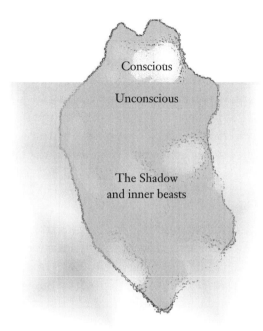

**Our psyche is like an iceberg—each person must identify and subdue his or her inner beasts which lurk beneath the surface.**

human being to go inside him/herself and face their inner beasts or unconscious forces, to confront them and subdue them. In this way, a person can take back their power, control it, and use it with conscious awareness.

The importance of this is reflected in another Greek myth— that of the Minotaur, a monster with the body of a man and the head of a bull who lived in the middle of a labyrinth and devoured all those who dared to confront him. Theseus finally succeeded in slaying the Minotaur and escaping from the labyrinth, thanks to the thread of Ariadne (in other words, with the help of love).

As homeopaths, we must play the role of Theseus for our patients—leading them through the labyrinth of their unconscious to find the Minotaur, and helping them to kill it. Only by doing so can they free themselves from the unconscious forces that contribute to disease and self-destruction. Without love, this task is impossible.

It is interesting to note that the name of the Minotaur incorporates the word *minos*, meaning minor or childhood. In other words, we are dealing here with unconscious forces whose roots are to be found in childhood.

The myth of the Minotaur persists today in the famous bullfights of Spain and Southern France. The toreador dresses in a shining suit—"clothes of light" which represent knowledge and wisdom. His mission is to go into the heart of the arena (representing the human body) and kill the bull (symbol of the blind powers of the unconscious, of blackness). Black is not a color, but rather the absence of light—a black cloth absorbs all light and reflects nothing. This is the quality of pure Ego. Just as life cannot exist without light or heat, neither can it exist in the presence of pure Ego.

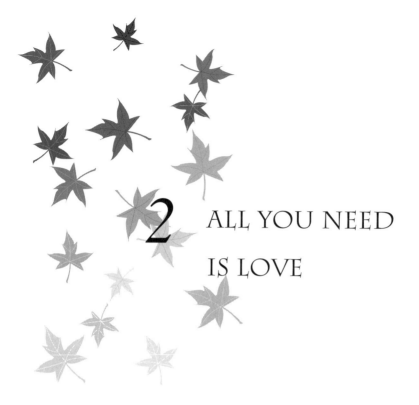

# 2    ALL YOU NEED IS LOVE

*Love is like the light that shows us the way out of our inner labyrinth.*

## THE THREE DIMENSIONS OF LOVE

When white light is directed through a prism, it splits into the three primary colors—blue, red, and yellow. It was again the Greeks who taught us that love also consists of three dimensions: *Eros, Philos,* and *Agape.*

## Eros

The first dimension, *Eros*, relates to the ego—to the "I" and its desire for personal pleasure. This kind of love is an indispensable first phase, as explained by Confucius and by Jesus Christ who said, "Love your neighbor *as you love yourself.*" We need to love ourselves first, love our ego, and so bring the billions of cells of which our physical body consists into a state of harmony and joy.

Each one of our cells could survive on its own. But each is also a specialist and plays a vital role for all the other cells. This is a community in which unemployment doesn't exist—the cells of the heart beat for the others, the cells of the feet walk for the others, the cells of the intestines digest for the others. A healthy body is like a utopian society, where all the members love each other and are in constant communication. There is no such thing as a useless, excluded, selfish, or lazy cell. What better example could human beings have than the microcosm of their own bodies?

## Philos

The second dimension of love, *Philos*, represents the "We," in which several individuals join together to form a group and love is exchanged between them. It is here that altruistic love starts to make an appearance, since a mother or father would run through fire to save their child.

The dimension of *Philos* starts with the couple and progressively expands to take in children, extended family, and the community. But even altruistic love such as this can become a shortcut to hell, dividing Serbs from Croats, Tutsis from Hutus, and so on. It is the source of all those tribal wars that have marked humanity since the beginning of time.

## Agape

The third dimension of love is *Agape*, which represents universal altruistic love. No longer do we refer to the "I" or the "We," but rather to the "One."

## THE GREAT MASTERS

These were people who attained *Agape,* or the third dimension of love, during their lifetimes, Jesus Christ being one example. Jesus did in fact describe himself as "the light of the world" and spoke of the Trinity residing within him. The three members of this Trinity—the Father, the Son, and the Holy Spirit—unite to form one, just as the three primary colors of yellow, red, and blue unite to form white light. Yellow is the color of the Sun or the Father, whose rays of light and heat give life to our planet. Red is the color of blood and therefore of the Son. Blue is the color of water—of the mother, the ocean, and Spirit.

## THE REMEDIES OF LOVE

Literally meaning "ignited by love," **Ignatia Amara** is the remedy for people suffering from disappointed or unhappy love. For them, the second dimension of love—that of the couple, of the "We"—is impossible to maintain because they want it to be all-consuming. They constantly hesitate between returning to the self-centered love of the "I" and progressing on to the third dimension of *Agape.*

Reputed to protect people from the plague, the St. Ignatius bean (from which the remedy is derived) was named by members of the Society of Jesus, in honor of their founder St. Ignatius Loyola (1491–1556). The characteristics of this remedy reflect the dilemma faced by St. Ignatius himself—a dilemma he solved by adopting the spiritual path.

Born a nobleman, St. Ignatius initially indulged his "I" by enjoying all the social pursuits and vanities of his time. He then fell in love with a woman whose social rank made any kind of relationship impossible, and the path to the "We" became forever barred to him. For her sake, he put himself through countless life-endangering acts of chivalry until, having injured himself during one of these exploits, he found himself at death's door. It was here that he discovered *Agape* or the third dimension of love, and chose to dedicate the rest of his life to the spiritual quest. This quest involved worshipping the Holy Trinity with such fervor that he would go into a state of ecstasy, his laughter alternating with tears of joy.

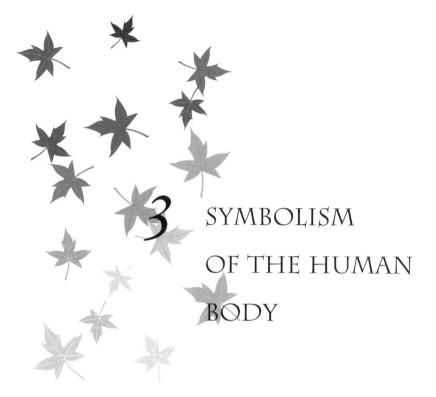

# 3 SYMBOLISM OF THE HUMAN BODY

The human body is like a vast temple, with the feet as its foundations and the head as its roof. When Jesus told his disciples that once the temple was destroyed it would take him three days to rebuild, he was alluding to the temple of his own body and to the three days between his crucifixion and resurrection.

If we relate the three dimensions of love to the physical body, then the feet represent the seed or the ego, the knees symbolize our progression to the "We," and the level of the hips are the third dimension of love. So, for example, the Bible tells of how Jacob spent a whole night wrestling with an angel, in other words with the forces of his own unconscious. He won the fight, but sustained a lifelong injury to his hip.

Only those who can rid their hearts of all hatred are able to reach this third dimension of *Agape*. This explains why Jesus advised someone who wished to pray, to first go and make friends with his enemies.

A young woman came to see me because her six-month-old baby spent every night screaming in its sleep. I thought it must be having nightmares and asked the mother whether she suffered from bad dreams. She told me that the night before, she had dreamt that her best friend crashed his car into another vehicle. I thought of **Anthracinum,** the anthrax nosode, which is an excellent remedy for boils and carbuncles and whose corresponding personality type has a fear of cars driving into it.

When I asked the mother if she had had any abscesses recently, she said that over the summer she had suffered from a carbuncle in her groin. I then asked whether she had been in an accident during the pregnancy. She revealed that, when seven months pregnant, a car had crashed in front of her. "I couldn't stop in time and went into it, and the safety belt pressed into my abdomen." I asked her what feelings she had had at that time and she replied, "Hatred for the woman who was driving the other car. I'd have killed her if she'd hurt my baby."

Boils and carbuncles are like little pockets of hatred, seething and literally "boiling over" with pus and anger. What this patient needed to do, for the sake of both herself and her baby, was to forgive the other driver.

However, true forgiveness can only be felt by those who have already confronted their own Shadow and inner beasts and have emerged triumphant from the labyrinth. These people understand that someone who commits a misdeed is like a child whose ego is being manipulated by the forces of his unconscious. This is why Jesus said, "Let the children come to me, and do not hinder them," because it is by identifying our children—the whims of our unconscious—that we can be healed.

Each of us prepares for our life on this planet during the nine months inside our mother, where we are bathed in infinite love. It is a self-centered love, since everything revolves around us, and is therefore pure ego—the first dimension. The purpose of human life is to leave the womb and progress through the second and then on to the third dimension of love.

This third dimension of love has been described by some who have had near-death experiences and saw a brilliant white light that they longed to go towards. Unfortunately, very few people experience this dimension of love in their earthly lifetimes. Only a few sages, mystics, and "blessed ones" receive brief revelatory flashes. These have been described as moments of ecstasy—the heart expands with a rush of pure love and the eyes weep in recognition and wonder, as the spirit perceives instantaneously that it is eternal, unique, and linked not just to every living creature, but to nature itself and the entire universe. The person realizes how much help and support each of us constantly receives, and longs to spread the good news to everyone he meets.

This is where things start to become complicated, since the person's enthusiasm often meets with a brick wall of resistance from his family, friends, and society. Even when he can show the fruits of his experience, in the form of newfound energies or skills, those around him remain unconvinced. What's more, his grand ideas of altruism and sharing tend to conflict with long-established systems, institutions, and egos which all have a vested interest in maintaining the *status quo*.

There is a saying in the South of France that captures this attitude perfectly: "Why give the donkey water when it isn't thirsty?" (*"On ne donne pas à boire l âne qui n'a pas soif."*) What this proverb is really referring to is people's readiness to increase their level of consciousness—only those who are already "thirsty" will make the change. People who have already reached this level of love and consciousness must therefore be patient and compassionate. They must let time do its work and, rather than trying to lead others, should simply guide them very gently—even when those they love seem to be marching straight towards a precipice. It is never too late for people to have a change of heart, mind, and direction. The donkey is bound to get thirsty one day!

## DUALITIES

The human body is divided into two by the diaphragm. The lower half relates to our connection to the Earth and symbolically to the mother, while the upper half relates to our yearning for the Heavens, symbolized by the father.

**Conium maculatum** is no longer able to draw up energy from the lower parts of his body to the upper parts, in order to attain higher consciousness. His lower limbs become paralyzed and he becomes old, senile, and lecherous.

We are also divided into two laterally. The right side of the body, which represents strength, reason, and rational thinking, relates to the father. The left side is artistic, intuitive, and sentimental and relates to the mother.

**Lycopodium** over-emphasizes his right side and then falls ill. He desires power and authority and identifies with the father—head of the family. His fear is that he will be unable to assert his authority and will instead be taken over by his own children.

**Lachesis,** on the other hand, places too much emphasis on the left side and falls ill from jealousy or emotional excitement. He can't bear for relationships to end, so tries to keep all his loved ones under tight control.

## THE BODY AND ITS SYMBOLS

### The Skin

As the body's primary protective barrier, the skin symbolizes the mother, whose womb formed our very first protective barrier against the outside world. Once outside the womb, we are exposed to the various challenges of our environment, such as cold, bacteria, and allergens, and we need to protect ourselves.

Eczema sufferers are expressing their regret at the loss of fusion with the mother. They want to be caressed and rubbed with soothing ointments. At the other extreme, someone with psoriasis is constantly shedding their skin—a metaphor for their attempt to break through the protective but stifling bond that their mother has placed around them.

In former times, someone with a skin condition was often told by his doctor to get down on his knees and thank God. Physicians knew that when a disease "came out" onto the skin, it was leaving the body and the patient would make a complete recovery. Successful homeopathic treatment often ends in a skin eruption, which should be left to resolve of its own accord, rather than pushing it back inside with cortisone ointments.

We cover our skin with clothing, which is symbolic of our external veneer. Doctors often ask their patients to undress so that they can examine them. This undressing represents the shedding of our outer façade in order to reveal the truth underneath.

**Platina** is the remedy for people who place too much importance on outer appearances and spend a fortune on expensive clothes.

Some people have white patches on their skin, which often date back to an unresolved grief **(Arsenicum album, Calcarea silica, Hura brasiliensis),** while *cafe au lait* marks are typical of **Carcinosin.**

Now that we have dealt with the body's outer covering, we can go on to each of its various parts and organs—starting with the feet and working upwards towards the head. This direction represents a journey from the past towards the future since, as every homeopath knows, diseases progress from the bottom up and from the outside in. Healing proceeds in the opposite direction—if a patient's last remaining symptom only affects his feet, we know that he is generally much better. Such symptoms are often the oldest and the last to disappear.

## The Feet

As we've already seen, the feet represent the seed, the foundation, the grounding force, and childhood.

As the practice of reflexology shows, the souls of the feet are covered with reflex points which correspond to each part of the body—the toes, for example, relating to the head and its various organs.

**Sulphur** is the remedy for people who want to "put their feet up" all the time and realize that, to do so, all they need is the wisdom to be content with what they have. A Sulphur person is a happy person, even if he's a tramp—his rags seem to him like robes of silk. He has an inner fire, like that of a volcano, which gives him the confidence to do exactly as he likes. His problem is that he doesn't feel any need to listen to others and take their opinions into account. He may well stink of sulphur, but since he can't smell it he doesn't care!

Phonetically, "Sulphur" is very similar to the word "suffer," and it is no coincidence that homeopaths consider this to be the deepest-acting remedy of Psora—the miasm of profound suffering. All humans feel this suffering, and Sulphur has been used to complete many a homeopathic cure.

## The Ankles

The ankle represents the weak point between foot and leg. We sprain our ankle (pull it out of alignment) when we fall out of alignment with those basic laws that form the structure and stability of life itself. One "false step" and we find ourselves paralyzed with pain.

A good remedy for repeated sprains is **Natrum carbonicum,** which is for people who are unable to reach a state of inner harmony and balance. Any balance they have is immediately destroyed by one of these ankle sprains, which occur as a result of the conflict between the ego (the foot) and the demands of altruistic love (the upper body), as each strains to move in a different direction.

**Rhus toxicodendron** is a remedy for acute sprains. People needing this remedy believe that movement is Life, so they move about too much, lose control, and end up hurting themselves.

## The Achilles Tendon

This is the weakest point of the human body. We rupture a tendon when we feel "torn between" several things—which one should we "tend" towards? We hesitate between the "I" of the feet and the "We" of the knees.

The Achilles tendon is joined to the twin muscles of the gastrocnemius soleus, which represent duality and **Anacardium**—the King of tendon remedies. In life, we each have to make choices, the most important being the choice between spirit and matter, ego and altruism. Man's weak point lies in this duality and his wavering between the two.

## The Knees

The knees represent the second dimension of love. Problems at this level are often symptomatic of a conflict between the demands of the ego and those of a love relationship.

A teenage boy came to me suffering from knee pains. When I asked him "What's her name?" he went bright red and asked me not to tell his parents!

Many of our best-known remedies have an affinity for the knees:

**Medorrhinum** has many love affairs and goes from one partner to another, reveling in his own sexuality and in the sexual act itself. He is too controlled by the demands of his ego—always wanting more and living in constant anticipation of his next sexual conquest. His problems lie in this succession of different "We's" that also make him prone to sexually transmitted diseases such as gonorrhea.

One of the key symptoms of Medorrhinum is a tendency to sleep on the front, in the knee-chest position like a toad. If the patient presents with warts or rheumatism, the symptoms will usually be focused around the knees.

**Iodum** patients are the ones who tear a ligament while playing football. As we will see later on, this remedy relates to our yearning for higher consciousness. Iodum is not satisfied with either the duality of the "We" or the vanity of the "I." He seeks the third dimension, but never stands still long enough to find it! Only through an enforced period of rest, as imposed by an injury, will he give himself the time to contemplate and thereby come closer to the spiritual dimension that he seeks.

## The Hips

The hips represent the gateway to the third dimension. Among those remedies with an affinity for the hips is **China (Cinchona officinalis** or Peruvian bark)—the very substance that led to Hahnemann's discovery of homeopathy. He had been translating a text by the British doctor Cullen, in which the latter described the malaria-like fevers of men working in warehouses where cinchona was stored.

Struck by the fact that cinchona was capable of treating those very same malarial fevers, Hahnemann decided to test the substance on himself and, after several days, started to experience the various symptoms described in his *Materia Medica*. This was to be the first homeopathic proving.

Apart from fever, the symptoms recorded by Hahnemann included exhaustion, anemia, and an excessive fear of animals. The China patient is like a tree that has had its bark removed. It loses its sap— its vital fluids—and becomes worn out. It is the remedy for people who want to get underneath their own shell in order to see and understand what lies within, but who lack the courage to confront their inner beasts.

China is also useful for those who have been exhausted by years of psychoanalysis—lost among the trees of their own symptoms, they are no longer able to "see the wood." They can't find the key to themselves, and it is significant that in daily life they are constantly losing their keys!

Following his experience with China, Hahnemann was able to "see the wood" of his own greater purpose and went on to complete more than a hundred more provings. His lifelong dedication to homeopathy gave him the knowledge and vitality to live a very long and productive life.

# THE ABDOMINAL AREA

## The Navel

Site of our former attachment to the mother, the navel is located right in the center of the abdomen and is symbolic of the ego. Someone who is completely self-absorbed is said to "contemplate his navel" or be "navel-gazing." An umbilical hernia signifies a desire to return to a fusional bond, like that which exists between a mother and baby.

**Abrotanum** experiences bleeding from the navel. He has never recovered from the cutting of his umbilical cord and has become energetically dependent on others. He's an "energy vampire" who drains everyone with whom he comes into contact.

## The Stomach

The stomach symbolizes our strength and courage to "swallow" those things that we find particularly indigestible, such as bad news.

Rigid and unforgiving, **Nitric acid** can't "digest" the injury done to him by his best friend and hates him for the rest of his life.

Literally "eaten up" with hatred, he eventually develops a stomach ulcer. Paradoxically, he may have a habit of eating indigestible things, such as soil and chalk.

## The Intestines

The intestines represent the meanders of our journey through the internal labyrinth, as we grapple with our Shadow self.

The person needing **Colocynthis** (the Bitter Cucumber) is unable to resolve his anger so instead expresses it physically, in the form of colic and abdominal spasms that "bend him in two."

**Arsenicum album** is a good remedy for acute episodes of diarrhea, which may be so exhausting that they endanger the patient's life. The key to this remedy lies in its fear of death and its doubts about what lies beyond. These doubts make the patient cling to the material world and he becomes mean and fastidious.

Constipation symbolizes a refusal to give. One of the main remedies for this is **Opium,** where all the vital functions become paralyzed following a major fright. The patient stops interacting with the outside world, cuts himself off from other people and from God, and finds himself in Hell—trapped inside his own inner labyrinth.

## The Kidneys

The kidneys are the higher-level equivalent of the feet and represent the internal seed, the seat of our ancestral power and energy. It is at this level that we are able to access our inner voice, in order to progress from the duality of the "We" to the Trinity located in the liver.

It is within the kidneys that we store fear. The fears we have of breaking our fusional bonds with others and of becoming autonomous effectively drain us of our primitive, ancestral energies.

**Phosphorus** is good for people who, unable to recover from a broken relationship, rapidly lose weight and energy. Literally "beside themselves," they feel more and more ungrounded and separated from their physical bodies and finally come down with nephritis. This remedy will resolve the illness and enable the patient to "get his feet back on the ground" and discover a more balanced kind of spirituality.

## The Pancreas

The pancreas is the powerhouse of the body, distributing the energy needed for creation (its name comes from the Greek *pan-kreas*— "all flesh"). Insulin produced in the pancreas enables sugar, the fuel, to penetrate every cell in the body and provide it with the energy it needs to live.

**Spongia** has an affinity for the pancreas. The basic characteristic of the person needing this remedy is that of the sponge, a marine animal that behaves like a plant. Rather than detaching itself and becoming independent, it clings to its rock and depends on the sea and currents to keep it alive. In the same way, the person needing Spongia fails to detach himself from the mother—he depends upon her completely, loses his autonomy and vegetates.

## The Spleen

Symbolic of nostalgia and regret for the past, the spleen is literally a dead end—a physiological cul-de-sac where the only way out is backwards.

**Capsicum** is the remedy for those who have been adversely affected by a move or migration. They start to put on weight, become insomniac, and suffer from mastoiditis (otitis in the area of the temporal bone—the bone relating to Time). What they are really yearning for is the paradise lost of their mother's womb.

## The Liver

The liver represents the gateway to higher levels—the passage from earth to heaven, via the diaphragm. The vein which carries nutrients to the liver is called the hepatic portal vein (portal coming from the Latin *porta* or "gate") and symbolizes the path to higher consciousness described in the Gospels: "The gate is narrow and the way is hard, and those who find it are few." We need to be true "livers," in other words live in faith, if we are to free ourselves from the material world.

**Chelidonium** refuses to see things as they are—instead of really living, he becomes bilious and suffers from liver pains. He is like Tobias, the blind man who was cured through the application of animal bile to his unseeing eyes. Chelidonium produces a yellow sap that resembles bile and is a very effective cure for warts when applied locally.

Lionel, an acquaintance, had led a mundane existence devoid of any particular aim, until a friend advised him to apply Chelidonium to the stubborn warts on his hands. Shortly afterwards, he suddenly became interested in spirituality and started to get involved in charities working in the Third World.

## THE ORGANS OF THE CHEST

### The Thymus

The thymus gland is the organ that enables us to distinguish between what is "me" and what is "not-me." It is the seat of our immunity, which is deficient in diseases such as AIDS.

**Kali iodatum** is often indicated in cases where the trachea is compressed by an overgrown thymus. The patient is subject to fixed ideas and opinions, from which he never wavers. He loses the ability to listen, understand, and recognize, and may even fail to recognize his own children. Here lies the key to those autoimmune diseases in which the body rejects its own organs—it is literally failing to "recognize its own."

## The Lungs

The lungs contain the breath of life and enable us to move from the womb to the outside world. Their constant rhythm of inspiration and expiration symbolizes the necessary alternation of give and take. Someone who has great ideas is said to be "inspired," while the Book of Genesis describes how Adam was created by God breathing onto clay.

**Ipecac** suffers from acute bouts of asthma or vomiting but has a clean tongue. He is someone who doesn't know what he wants and gets everything the wrong way around—he retains the stale air that he should release, and vomits the food that he should digest.

Coughing is often due to a feeling of being "suffocated" by those around us. Children who have spent the entire summer free to play and do as they please often start coughing when they have to return to the restrictions of school and life in a community. Coughing can also be a means of expressing regret or grief, as in the dry spasmodic cough of **Ignatia** following separation from a loved one due to death or divorce.

## The Pleura

This transparent membrane surrounds and protects the lungs and respiratory apparatus. It is symbolic of home, which shelters and protects us and which we don't want to leave.

**Bryonia** is struck down with pleuropneumonia at the prospect of going on holiday or to summer camp. Bryonia is a wild hop whose enormously long roots burrow deep into the ground.

## The Ribs

The ribs form a protective cage around all of the delicate organs of the chest. In the Old Testament, God creates Eve using one of Adam's ribs. So the rib symbolizes the person at our side—the relationship with our partner.

**Kalmia latifolia** is useful for fractured ribs. Psychologically, it is for people who like to play the matchmaker—they want to feel like they're indispensable and that the whole world revolves around them. They want to keep everyone in a cage.

**Cactus grandiflorus** is a flower that blooms at night, when nobody can see it. The Cactus child suffers from asthma, with a sensation as if his ribcage were gripped in a vice. He can't bear to be watched doing his homework, since this makes him feel like a caged animal at the zoo.

## Blood

Blood is oxygenated in the lungs and consists of red blood cells that have no nucleus. This lack of a nucleus relates to our ability to separate ourselves from the mother, with the help of the father.

**Natrum muriaticum**'s suffering is caused by his father's rejection and disappearance from his life. There is "bad blood" between the child and his father, which may eventually manifest itself as a blood disease such as leukemia.

Hemoglobin contains iron, which serves to fix the oxygen. **Ferrum metallicum** is the remedy for people with anemia who are no longer able to "fix" on any objective and become "bloodless." This remedy will enable them to discover their innate "iron will."

## The Heart

The heart is master of the circulatory system. It is the only organ that works continuously from the start of life, tirelessly distributing blood to all the other organs just as the sun sends out its golden rays to all forms of life.

Both the heart and gold are symbolic of the father's role and ultimately of God—the source of life itself.

**Aurum metallicum** is the remedy for those who, on some level, want to play a God-like role on earth. They seek wealth so that they can then distribute it to others and therefore become the source of everything. Unfortunately, in order to do this, they have to break the laws of the one true God and may even go so far as to kill. They are then wracked with a terrible sense of guilt and remorse, which drives them to commit suicide or develop a fatal heart disease.

## THE UPPER LIMBS

### The Fingers

These symbolize the fingers of God, pointing us in the right direction. The ten fingers are the Ten Commandments that are indispensable to a community's survival (thou shalt not kill, neither shalt thou commit adultery, neither shalt thou steal, etc).

The necessity of the Ten Commandments is the central issue for the person in need of the remedy **Digitalis,** which is Latin for "finger" or "digit." For him, the Ten Commandments make life dull—pleasure is forbidden and it's his heart that suffers! It is the remedy for people who seem allergic to work and effort, especially when it's imposed on them.

### The Hands

These represent potential creativity and therefore the future. We need to "grab our life with both hands" and act now, rather than constantly putting things off until tomorrow. The handshake is used to seal friendships and agreements—so a hand covered in eczema or warts symbolizes an unwillingness to become involved with others.

### The Wrists

The wrists represent human strength (in direct opposition to the ankles, which represent human weakness).

**Calcarea carbonica** may develop a synovial cyst on the wrist. He is unable to shake off the sense of his own weakness that explains his numerous fears—including a fear of animals.

## The Elbow

We lift our elbow in order to either hit others or defend ourselves. **Bromium** has eczema around the elbows because when he's on land he feels the need to protect himself from attack. He dreams of getting back on his boat and returning to the sea.

**Agaricus** has tendonitis of the elbow—he has too much energy, hits too hard, and his body suffers the consequences.

**Phosphorus** presents with psoriasis around the elbows—being a gentle soul, he doesn't want to hit anyone.

## The Shoulders

As in the legend of Atlas, our shoulders bear the weight of the world. We have to "put our shoulder to the wheel" if we want to make it!

**Calcarea phosphorica** is a near-specific for arthritis of the shoulder joint due to calcification. This joint forms a cross between the vertical line of the spinal cord and the horizontal line of the outstretched arms. To Calcarea phosphorica, then, the world seems terribly unfair—he feels he has to "bear his cross." As a child, his reluctance to grow up causes him to suffer from "growing pains."

In her job as a social worker, Anne-Laure was constantly having to "shoulder" situations of extreme poverty, in both the material and the emotional senses. By the time she was forty, she had already been diagnosed with arthritis of the shoulder joint.

**Oleum jecoris aselli** has a corresponding affinity for ankylosing spondylitis. This is a disease that affects the sacro-iliac joint—the horizontal/vertical cross of the lower body.

## The Thyroid

Regulator of body temperature and growth, the thyroid's role is just as important as that of the liver in our progress towards spirituality.

**Iodum** (iodine) was the mineral that enabled fish to leave the water and survive on land, since it is the driving force of catabolism—the burning up of flesh in order to produce heat. While thermoregulation can be a slow process when in the water, in air we have to adapt to rapid variations in temperature. Symbolically, the progression from water to land represents the progression from that original, all-consuming bond between mother and child towards a more altruistic love in which each respects the other's individuality. Iodum refuses to make this leap, tries to return to a former state and develops thyroid problems or else otitis media with effusion—a kind of otitis which forces him to hear everything through water, just as though he were still in the womb.

## The Larynx

The larynx is modulator of the voice, which represents the ability to speak our truth. There is a saying "use it or lose it," and when we lose our voice it is because we have stopped speaking our truth. In certain situations, when we don't know how to react, we are said to be "rendered speechless"—this is the source of many an acute or chronic sore throat.

**Aconite** loses his voice following a violent shock and goes into an acute attack of laryngitis at 11:00 P.M.

**Spongia** is aggravated by wet weather and sea breezes. Like a sponge, dependent on the tides and currents of the sea, he is unable to leave his mother and speak his own truth. He is suffocated and starts to experience breathing problems.

**Hepar sulphuricum** has lost touch with his own truth and sense of direction. He believes that the world is corrupt and should be set on fire so that things can become clearer. He develops a hoarse, barking cough.

**Calcarea bromata** feels in danger in his own home. The people who should protect him (his parents) have proved incapable of doing so, and teething brings on laryngitis.

**Arum triphyllum** ("Jack in the Pulpit") has a duotone voice. He is unable to choose his own truth and decide which path to take, and wavers between two "voices."

**Calcarea sulphurica** loses his voice from jealousy, when everyone's attention turns towards his newborn baby brother or sister.

**Calcarea carbonica** is afraid of everything—every truth and every path seems fraught with danger. He suffers from chronic laryngitis and sore throats.

**Cuprum** is another remedy with an affinity for the larynx and is for people who don't feel up to speaking and following their truth. They may be born with laryngomalacia (abnormal softening of the larynx due to decalcification) causing harsh, difficult breathing.

## The Mouth

Source of the word, the mouth is a symbolic combination of the male and female sexual organs, with its hollow opening and phallic tongue. The resulting "child"—the word—is sacred, because it results from a kind of immaculate conception. Correspondingly, the speaker of the word becomes like God in his ability to create this sacred "child" unilaterally. This is in complete contrast to the lower body, where we are sexual beings and only possess half of what is needed to create a human child.

Stammering reflects a person's inability to articulate the right word—the flow of speech is interrupted and words are repeated spasmodically. **Mercurius solubilis** stammers in his attempt to speak rapidly enough to bamboozle his listeners. This is a reminder of the remedy's namesake, Mercury—the precocious child who, initiated by the gods as their messenger to mankind, was tempted to change the messages to his own ends. Patients needing this remedy give themselves away by their bad breath, profuse salivation, and constant stammering.

**Lilium tigrinum** is frightened of saying something that's not true. One day she stops talking altogether and goes into a state of constant physical activity. This remedy is for people who would like to be sole creators and thereby retain their purity.

## The Nose

Situated right in the middle of the face, the nose's position is analogous to that of the spinal cord and is a well-known symbol for the penis. The male organ penetrates, and someone who follows their nose follows their intuition and therefore penetrates to the heart of the matter. In the same way, someone with a blocked nose has lost touch with what is important in life. Intuition is one of the essential qualities of man, counterbalanced as it is by reason and intellect. We should learn to follow our nose and listen to our intuition.

**Plumbum** can no longer sense or feel anything. Everything becomes heavy and burdensome, like a lead weight.

**Colchicum**'s sense of smell is so acute that the smell of cooking makes him vomit. These are people for whom good manners are all important—they yearn to be aristocrats and to have a life "above stairs," well away from the smells of the kitchen and other mundane aspects of life.

## The Sinuses

These are closely linked to the nasal cavities. The maxillary sinuses enable us to locate ourselves in space, the frontal sinuses in time.

**Mezereum** feels disorientated following a move—he has lost all his points of reference and develops chronic inflammation of both the maxillary sinuses.

**Thuja,** meanwhile, has problems with the frontal sinuses—he would like to be in control of everything but can't control the passage of time.

## The Ears

The ears enable us to listen to the outside world and relate to others. In addition, the internal ear and its labyrinthine structure enable us to locate ourselves spatially and keep our balance. The internal ear houses the meanderings of the "I."

The ears are to the head what the feet are to the lower body and the kidneys to the torso—they represent the seed within. Acupuncturists consider the external ear to be representative of the whole body, and they manipulate it accordingly.

**Tellurium** suffers from eczema on the external ear, caused by acrid discharge from chronic otitis. He is a hypersensitive person and his symptoms can often be traced back to an insensitive remark that threw him completely "off balance."

**Conium maculatum**'s hearing improves when the wax is removed from his ears. He spends a great deal of time and effort in the pursuit of higher consciousness but has forgotten that the most important thing is to listen to others. Even looking to the side—in other words, at other people—makes him feel dizzy.

## The Eyes

The eyes enable us to see the world and are at the same time "mirrors of the soul." Recently, one of my patients who comes from a Jewish family told me, *"Nous avons des problèmes d'yeux dans la famille."* ("We have eye problems in our family.")

However, what I heard was the phonetically identical: *"Nous avons des problèmes Dieu dans la famille."* ("We have God problems in our family!") I asked her if her family was religious, and she explained that they had been atheists ever since their internment in the Nazi concentration camps during the last war. Refusing to progress along the road towards higher consciousness, they were expressing their spiritual suffering through recurrent eye problems. These were resolved with a few doses of Opium.

**Opium** doubts the existence of Heaven and falls prey to all kinds of fears and guilt-feelings.

## The Hair

The hair represents our strength, beauty, and power, and in particular our sexual power. Samson lost his power when his hair was cut.

**Phosphoricum acidum** feels wiped out by sorrow following a death or bad news, and his hair starts to fall out by the handful.

**Chelidonium** falls prey to spiritual doubts and develops a bald patch on the crown, just like a monk. It is through this part of the head that we connect energetically with higher levels of consciousness.

Sometimes the hair goes prematurely gray—always a useful symptom for the homeopath! People needing **Lycopodium** would like their hair to turn white, since they see this as a sign of age and wisdom.

## The Brain

Seat of the intellect, the brain can be either a help or a hindrance, since it often leads us to over-complicate matters. The two cerebral hemispheres are the source of our duality. The left side, which controls the right side of the body, is the seat of reason and rationality, of the masculine principle, while the right side controls the left side of the body and is responsible for feelings, relationships and the feminine principle. The two hemispheres are linked via the *corpus callosum* and separated by the *falx cerebri*.

**Naja** is for people whose symptoms reflect a lack of communication between the two hemispheres of the brain. If a Naja commits suicide, he will do it by splitting his head in two with an axe.

## The Meninges

The names of the three meninges that surround the brain—the *pia mater*, the *arachnoid*, and the *dura mater*—are highly significant. *Pia mater* is Latin for "pious mother"—the woman who had enough love and faith to let us go and give us our autonomy; the *arachnoid* ("spider") enclosed us in its inescapable web of bonded love; while the *dura mater* ("hard mother") didn't love us enough.

Symptoms affecting any of the three meninges are thus always related in some way to issues with the mother or mother figure.


## DREAMS

In conclusion, we can see that the symbolism of diseased organs enables us to understand the unconscious forces at work. Another method for understanding illness is psychoanalysis and in particular dream analysis, since the unconscious expresses itself in dreams via symbols and metaphors.

For example, when I was a medical student one of my friends told me he was undergoing psychoanalysis for various problems that he couldn't understand. We were at that time receiving anatomy lessons on the pelvic area, and our lecturer, a surgeon, had told us of the danger that butchers run of injuring their femoral artery through a slip of the knife. This explained why they often wore several aprons. That night, my friend dreamt he was a butcher and that he cut his femoral artery—in French, his *artère fémorale*. Telling this to his psychoanalyst, the latter—who hadn't said a word for weeks — suddenly sat up and said, *"Fémorale—fait moral!"* While the two sound almost identical in French, their meanings are completely different, since a *fait moral* is a "moral offense!" Suddenly, my friend remembered having witnessed just such a "moral offense" as a child, which he had never managed to assimilate. The memory had remained in his unconscious and then expressed itself in his dream through a phonetic metaphor.

The power of psychoanalysis lies in the fact that it operates via the word itself, making it one of the royal roads to healing. "Just say the word and he will be healed," said the Centurion to Jesus. The right word can act like a sword, penetrating to the very heart of the patient's problem. In practice, though, psychoanalysis has its limits because the practitioner doesn't take into account physical signs and symptoms that would enable him to speed up the process.

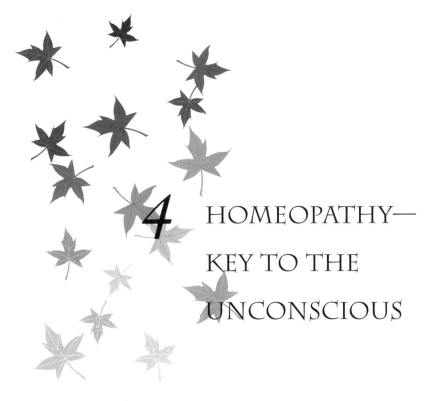

# 4 HOMEOPATHY— KEY TO THE UNCONSCIOUS

Homeopathy provides us with another key, both to the unconscious and to the language of the physical body.

The homeopathic method is based on the results of remedy provings. Healthy volunteers take potentized dilutions of a certain substance for several days running until they start to experience symptoms. These proving symptoms are carefully noted down, using the exact words of the prover. The number and quality of symptoms will depend upon both the substance used and the sensitivity of the individual. At the end of the proving, all the symptoms are recorded and classified in the homeopathic *Materia Medica*. Some of these symptoms result from the primary action of the substance itself, while others result from the secondary reaction of the prover.

Proving symptoms may be physical or mental. Dreams are considered to be particularly important, since they reflect the basic essence of the substance and are highly specific.

The truth of this was demonstrated to me through the remedy **Muriaticum acidum.** It was Hahnemann himself who conducted the original proving of hydrochloric acid, and he and his colleagues recorded nearly 600 symptoms, including that of "Difficult, disturbed sleep; on the fourth day dreamed that his mother died."

Some two centuries later, a seven-year-old boy was brought to my clinic by his desperate mother. She told me that her son was constantly ill, with one bout of bronchitis after another. Looking through his medical records, I noticed that the boy had twice suffered from hemorrhoids, which is very unusual for a child. A glance at *Kent's Repertory* gives just one remedy for this symptom—Muriaticum acidum.

Though comparatively young, the boy's mother was anxious, tired, and prematurely wrinkled. I asked her how she felt herself, and she told me that she'd slept badly for years due to a recurrent nightmare which woke her up every night and prevented her from going back to sleep. On further questioning, she revealed that the dream she had was of her mother dying! Looking in Hahnemann's *Materia Medica Pura* and finding this to be one of the proving symptoms of Muriaticum acidum, I felt a shiver go up my spine!

I then asked the woman about her mother, and she told me that she had died of tuberculosis when she herself was seven. They were living in Morocco at the time, but then moved back to France. One generation on, her son's recurrent bronchitis and horrendous coughing were forcing this woman to constantly relive her own mother's death. I prescribed Muriaticum acidum for them both—the son's bronchitis disappeared and the mother started to sleep again.

I concluded from this experience that the remedy Muriaticum acidum relates to anxieties about losing one's mother. Could it be that the nerve impulses linked to such emotions use hydrochloric acid as a transmitter?

Some time later, a male patient asked me to give him something for painful hemorrhoids that had resisted all kinds of treatment for three weeks. Noting his anxious expression, I asked him how his mother was. He blanched, then told me that three weeks earlier his mother had been diagnosed with terminal cancer. While this patient didn't feel able to say "My mother's dying," he could tell me "I've got hemorrhoids," and the homeopathic process enabled us to link his physical symptom with those anxieties which, until then, he had felt unable to express.

Another patient was in despair at the sight of her twenty-five-year-old son's slide into alcoholism. Needless to say, many different techniques had been tried over the years to help him kick his addiction, which was destroying the whole family and ruining his life. When I asked about the pregnancy, his mother told me that it had been very traumatic due to the death of her own mother around that time. I therefore prescribed a single dose of Muriatic acidum 15C, which put her son on the road to recovery. Having experienced the grief of losing a mother while still in the womb, this young man had felt unable to leave his own mother and become an adult.

As detailed in my first book *The Spirit of Homeopathic Medicines*, hundreds more homeopathic remedies have been studied in this way, enabling us to trace physical illnesses back to unexpressed words and feelings. "In the beginning was the Word … and the Word became flesh" as the Gospel of St. John tells us. In the beginning there are words, and these words are transmuted into physical illnesses. When words remain unspoken, they are suppressed into the unconscious and can act like a curse affecting several generations, as they get handed down from parent to child.

This transmutation of the word into flesh is easily explained by recent discoveries in the field of neurophysiology. When speech vibrates against the ear, nerve impulses are transmitted to the brain. While these messages travel along the nerve in the form of an electric current, it is chemicals that enable them to jump from one nerve to the next. These chemical substances in the brain are closely related to those found in the world around us, and it is these same substances that are used in homeopathy. The *most* similar remedy

—the *similimum*—relates to that chemical which made the first neurological link following speech. This sets up a domino effect of chemical reactions, extending down through every level and out to every part of the body. The endocrine system is just one of the levels affected.

Psychoanalysts operate at the level of the word, while classical homeopaths try to identify the similimum corresponding to that first chemical neurotransmitter. Other homeopaths work more on the periphery and the symptoms created by these successive chemical reactions, while allopaths try to correct their organic manifestations.

## HAHNEMANN'S THREE MIASMS

Having developed the theory of homeopathy, Hahnemann went on to identify the three basic miasms responsible for chronic disease. Looking at these three miasms today, we can see that they correspond very closely to the three dimensions of love, as well as to Freud's three stages of psychosexual development.

Hahnemann attributed the first miasm, Psora, to scabies or "the itch." It represents lack, destitution, cold, and hunger, but also the sufferings of the "I" and Freud's oral stage.

The second miasm, Sycosis, was attributed to gonorrhea and represents excess, power, and lack of control, as well as the "We" and the anal stage of Freud.

The third miasm, Syphilis, represents destruction, jealousy, murder, and Freud's Oedipus complex, plus progression to the "One"—the third dimension of love.

A person's psychological development is influenced by these three forces from the moment of his or her conception, when the gametes of the father fuse with those of the mother, right up until the end of life.

**Infinite love**
Mother/child
Egoism

**Infinite love**
Altruism

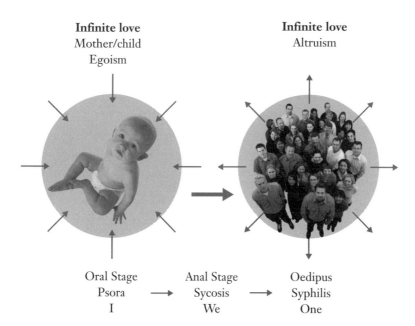

Oral Stage    Anal Stage       Oedipus
Psora   ⟶   Sycosis    ⟶   Syphilis
I                      We                  One

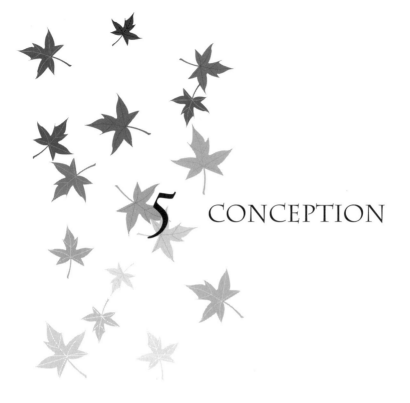

# 5 CONCEPTION

Most people in the world have no problem conceiving—on the contrary, the cities of developing countries are overflowing with thousands of unwanted children. The overriding problem on our planet today is more one of contraception.

Increasingly, though, couples in developed countries find it impossible to conceive and have to turn towards modern medical techniques for help. In such cases, we need to find out whether—on an unconscious level—both partners really want a child.

**Sepia** is unable to come to terms with the idea of becoming a mother. She prefers to remain childless, still a little girl on some level, with her partner acting as a symbolic replacement for her inaccessible father.

**Lycopodium** doesn't want children since these would restrict his freedom and take up all his energy. He has more important things to do—such as developing his career.

Martine thought she couldn't have children, but after a single dose of Lycopodium 15C she became pregnant. However, in the fifth month of pregnancy, she started to experience premature contractions. I saw her again, and, in order to confirm my belief that she needed another dose of Lycopodium, asked her if she liked oysters. "Oh no," she replied, "I hate the thought of having something alive inside me!" Lycopodium 30C enabled her to bring her pregnancy to term without further problems.

**Platina** can't bear the fact that pregnancy would distort her body and change people's attitudes towards her, while pale, anemic **Ferrum metallicum** doesn't have the inner strength needed to create a baby.


## THE MOMENT OF CONCEPTION

The ultimate climax of physical lovemaking occurs when the two gametes, male and female, unite. Several billion spermatozoa are left to fight it out in the ruthless struggle to penetrate a single egg. Recent studies have shown that the ovum favors the sperm cell whose genetic code is most different from its own. In other words, this microscopic egg has the wisdom needed to ensure optimal genetic inheritance for the resulting child.

In Greek mythology, Metis was the goddess renowned for her wisdom, and the same word "Métis" is used to describe a person of mixed parentage. Closely related genes need to be kept apart in order to avoid the risk of genetic defects, which explains why opposites often attract. Society's prohibition of incest is therefore based on sound biological principles.

In spite of these protective measures, no child is ever perfect. In addition to its innate talents and positive characteristics, he or she will also inherit certain flaws that will need to be dealt with later in life.

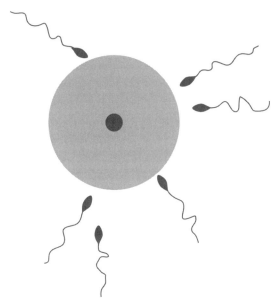

**The sperm cell whose genetic code differs most from that
of the ovum is the one allowed to enter.**

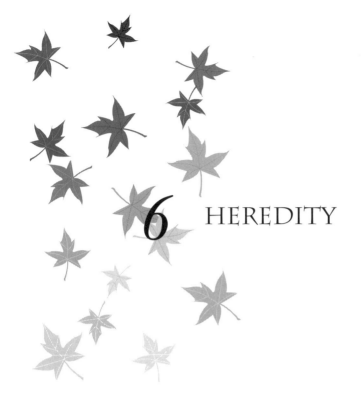

# 6 HEREDITY

The chromosomes carry our physical heredity—a heredity that can sometimes be a burden, as in cases such as hemophilia, cystic fibrosis, muscular dystrophy, and Down's syndrome.

But researchers like Serge Tisseron (*Tintin et les Secrets de Famille* 1990) and Anne Ancelin-Schützenberger (*Aïe, mes Aïeux* 1993) have demonstrated how each of us also possesses a psychological heredity in which veritable family sagas are played out over several generations.

In some families, for example, everyone has a serious accident at around the same age, which is always due to some apparently coincidental outside event. It is no accident that the Hebrew word for "chance" also means "help" or "aid."

People needing **Sulphuricum acidum** often inherit this running theme of the accident. Driven by unconscious motives, they act recklessly and repeat the same kind of scenario generation after generation.

Sometimes, one generation of a family is so strongly affected by a particular trauma that the memory of it is transmitted to successive generations. Eventually, the memory is driven so deep into the unconscious that those who inherit it are unable to understand the reason for their suffering.

Feelings of this sort can become the driving force for a unique level of creativity, as was the case with Hergé—inventor of the famous Tintin cartoon books. The purpose of Hergé's books was to gradually reveal his own family secret, and he identified himself with Captain Haddock and the search for *The Secret of the Unicorn.*

Hergé's family saga began with a nobleman's clandestine affair with one of his servants, the cook. Having become pregnant with twins, the cook was hurriedly married off to Rémi, the gardener.

Once born, the twin brothers were particularly well cared for, but the silk clothing given to them by their real father made them a laughing stock in the servant's quarters. These brothers were to become the Thompson Twins of Hergé's cartoons—no matter how hard they tried to disguise themselves, they were always instantly recognizable for who they really were.

Hergé (an anagram of R.G.—Rémi George) was the child of one of these twins, in other words the nobleman's illegitimate grandson. In his cartoons, Hergé's alter ego Captain Haddock rediscovers his own nobility (he is the Knight Hadoque), his castle of Moulinsard, plus the family jewels, but swears never to reveal the secret to anyone.

Some of the most harrowing family secrets are linked to a death. I once had an eight-year-old boy brought to me whose father had died one night of a heart attack. The boy had immediately been sent to stay with his grandmother, but she couldn't bring herself to tell him his father was dead. The next morning, the boy woke up covered in urticaria and the grandmother, a country woman, fed him with nettle soup which rapidly cured him.

Hearing this story, I realized that nettle—**Urtica urens**—must be the remedy that relates to the death of the father. The plant is covered with tiny hairs that make the skin itch, just like the bristles on Daddy's chin when he kisses his child at bedtime. Urtica urens is already well-known in homeopathy as a remedy for increasing breast milk production, as well as for curing urticaria and seafood allergies, but not a single mental symptom had been identified from the provings.

One day, I was called to see one of the newborns in a maternity hospital. The mother asked me for something to increase her milk, which had dried up, and my prescription of Urtica urens 7C quickly solved the problem. When I next saw the mother, several days later, I asked her what had happened on the day her milk dried up. She told me that she'd received a shock that morning, because when her baby was brought to her he was "all yellow" (he had slight jaundice). I then asked about her own father, and she explained that he had died several years earlier from liver cancer. "One day, he just turned all yellow; three weeks later, he was dead." The sight of her jaundiced son had unconsciously reminded this woman of her father's death, and her milk had dried up.

Some time later, I saw a child who was suffering from otitis media with effusion. His father was asthmatic and he was the eldest child—the one who usually takes on the father's issues. (The second child usually takes on the mother's issues, while from the third child onwards anything can happen!)

I asked the father how long he'd had asthma, and he told me that as a baby he'd suffered from eczema, which had been "cured" with cortisone ointments. His eczema had started when he suddenly had to be weaned off breast milk, which had dried up on the day his mother learned of her own father's sudden death.

This story is just one example of how a single theme can spread its disease-causing effects over several generations. Running alongside the individual unconscious (of the self or the "I") is another *family* unconscious, of the "We." This family unconscious is filled with all kinds of secrets and stories which are transmitted both *across* members of the same generation and *down* through successive generations. This helps to explain why people from different generations of the same family can benefit from the same remedy.

In the same way, there is also a wider collective unconscious—the unconscious of the third dimension or of the "One"—which affects the whole of society, as described by Jung. The collective unconscious is a significant factor in epidemics such as influenza, when the majority of those afflicted will need the same homeopathic remedy.

Probably the worst, and frequently the most hidden, kind of suffering occurs after the death of a child. The remedy for this is **Hura brasiliensis**—the milky sap or latex that is called Assacu by the Brazilians of Hura.

People who need this remedy express their suffering through various joint and limb problems, such as rheumatoid arthritis, and it is interesting to note that the blood of people suffering from rheumatoid arthritis has the coagulative properties of latex. The love of Hura brasiliensis towards others is also like a piece of elastic—the more the loved one tries to move away, the stronger Hura brasiliensis pulls the person back. The moment of crisis comes when the elastic breaks. Having experienced the death of their child as a sudden rupture in the bond of love, these people express their pain through the elastic fibers of their physical body (i.e. in the joints).

Hura brasiliensis is also a remedy for leprosy. People suffering from leprosy are outcasts, and in former times this disease often presented the only means for a person to escape from a suffocating relationship or bond. Excluded from their community, they could finally get away from their overbearing parents and live their lives elsewhere. Hura can also be considered in cases of vitiligo after the death of a child, when one family member becomes so over-possessive of his other relatives that he practically strangles them with love.

When parents can't come to terms with a child's death, they sometimes give their next baby the same Christian name—thereby transferring all the emotional charge of the death onto the newborn. One patient told me he'd named his son Gerard after his grandfather, who had looked after him when he was little since his parents owned a business and were always working. The grandfather had died suddenly, and he never got over it.

The remedy to think of in cases such as this is **Calcarea silica.** These are people who fail to break their ties with the dead, even going to far as to speak to them every day and tell them their problems and secrets.

A ten-year-old girl was brought to me because she was still having to sleep in her mother's bed. The two had never spent a night apart since the daughter's birth, and various medical and psychotherapeutic treatments had been tried in vain.

Knowing that psychoanalysts consider sleep to be a "little death," and sleep problems to signal an unresolved death, I asked the mother if there had been any particularly traumatic deaths in her own family. She told me that at the age of fifteen she had lost her father in an accident. When I asked her where her father was now, she pointed to the empty space on her right and said, "He's there. He never leaves my side."

Another five-year-old patient refused to go to sleep, saying he was scared because every night a man would come into his room. The mother turned to me and said, "My father died when I was six months pregnant." Everything improved after both mother and son had received a dose of Calcarea silica 30C. The mother said to me, "The night after we took the remedy, the man left. You thought it was my father as well, didn't you?"

## BACK TO HAHNEMANN'S MIASMS

The three main miasmatic trends, as Hahnemann called chronic disease, are transmitted hereditarily and can be identified from the patient's personal and family history.

Allergies, eczema, and nutritional problems tend towards Psora, with the forsaken feelings of **Psorinum** or the desire of **Tuberculinum** to leave its body and escape this cruel world.

Sycosis represents the tumor diathesis, with **Carcinosin** being the main remedy for families who keep their secret very closely guarded and never reveal it to anyone—"There are some things you just don't talk about." These are people who never express their feelings in order to avoid offending others and finally develop cancer, which is the loss of cellular differentiation.

Other sycotic conditions include hypertension, obesity, and diabetes, which tend towards **Medorrhinum** with its constant anxiety about the future at the expense of the present—the only thing that is real and eternal.

Finally, the Syphilitic miasm is indicated in families that are prone to genetic deformities, circulatory diseases, alcoholism, and suicide. **Syphilinum,** for example, develops a sudden mania for hand-washing, as though to cleanse himself after committing a crime.

Should we be angry with our ancestors for the various flaws and miasms they have handed down to us? Certainly not! *"Similia Similibus Curentur,"* or "like cures like," so we chose to be born into a family whose level of vibration corresponded with our own. We knew this would enable us to confront those very issues and problems we still needed to resolve in our journey towards infinite love. Even if they make life seem unfair or cruel, it is these problems that show us the way.

The situation is slightly different in the case of adopted children whose origins are unknown. Such children often need **Magnesia carbonica,** as they experience dreams of being "forced to marry against their will." In most Western societies, marriage is considered such an intimate and personal affair that the idea of it as a convenient arrangement between the families of two people who don't even know each other seems strange. And yet arranged marriages have always existed and still take place throughout the world. The same kind of scenario occurs in adoption, when a child is suddenly handed over to two people he doesn't know and with whom he has none of the close bonds which are built during those nine months in the womb.

Another clinical case gave me much insight into cases of adoption. As a pediatrician concerned with abandoned "problem" children, I came across the case of a child born with herpetic encephalitis. Since this disease usually causes permanent damage, nobody wanted to adopt the child. However, the baby was developing normally, so I discussed his case with a couple who had been trying to adopt for several years. (While adoption is a very difficult procedure for those wanting so-called "normal" children, it is usually much quicker when the couple is willing to adopt child with a disability.)

The couple hesitated for a while, then, when the baby reached nine months, decided to adopt. It was love at first sight between the adoptive father and the baby. As soon as the new family arrived home, the baby crawled through the apartment into the study and pointed to a book on the shelf. The following week, the father had to go away on business for a few days. On his return, the baby once again led him into the study and pointed to the same book.

The book in question was a novel by Dostoevsky—the only Russian book that the couple owned. When I asked the father if there was any Russian blood in his family, his face lit up as he exclaimed, "My grandfather was a Russian surgeon in exile during the Revolution. He got my Parisian grandmother pregnant, then disappeared without a trace, totally abandoning them both."

Perhaps this time it was the grandfather's turn to be abandoned and then rescued by his very own offspring....

So the law of "like cures like" can also be seen to apply in cases of adoption. When treating an adopted child, we should never fail to inquire about its adoptive parents' family history.

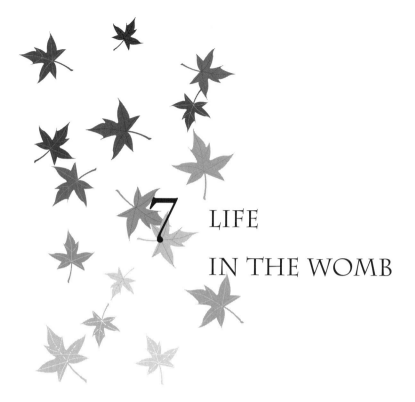

# 7 LIFE IN THE WOMB

## TIME AND SPACE

We tend to have an idealistic image of life in the womb: kept warm, fed and oxygenated, the only effort we have to make is to grow. Between the unicellular stage and birth, time is infinite. In reality, time does not pass in a linear fashion throughout life—the older we are, the faster it goes, as we all discover at some point! So it follows that time in the womb is at the opposite extreme— when the embryo still consists of just a few cells, time expands and stretches to become infinite.

Space also changes dramatically during our nine months in the womb, from being practically infinite (relative to the micro-scopic zygote) to highly restrictive at the end of gestation. This eventual lack of space is undoubtedly one of the reasons for our sudden decision to "move out."

However, even in this mini-paradise of the mother's womb, life is far from perfect since any event that occurs during pregnancy hits the fetus hardest of all. Whatever happens to the mother is also experienced by her unborn child, not just physically via the placenta, but on an energetic level as well.

## POSITIVE TRANSFUSIONS

Bathed in a soft red light, soothed by the muffled regular beat of the mother's heart, the fetus senses the positive emotions of its mother when she sees a breathtaking scenery, looks at a beautiful flower, or listens to Mozart. It was the Greeks who first thought of placing pregnant women in beautiful, calm surroundings in order that they could imbibe feelings of harmony and joy. They hoped this would produce relaxed, intelligent, and well-balanced children. By the same token, the Tziganes of Hungary play their violins over a woman's bulging abdomen in order to ensure that the baby becomes a musician.

## NEGATIVE TRANSFUSIONS

In our modern-day world, negative experiences occur on a daily basis during a woman's pregnancy. A child of six was once brought to me because he was waking every night at 3:00 A.M. and suffered from frequent bouts of copious diarrhea. What struck me during the consultation was how incredibly agitated he was. For me, his agitation was an expression of his fear of death, the remedy for which is **Arsenicum album.** I prescribed the same remedy for him and his mother, who was dressed in black, seemed very nervous and fastidious, and suffered from recurrent frontal sinusitis.

The frontal sinuses are located in the area identified by Hindus as the "Third Eye" and represent the doorway to the third dimension—that of spirituality. Sinusitis expresses the conflict triggered at this stage of a person's development, when a choice must be made between the material and the spiritual worlds.

During this first consultation, the mother had told me that her pregnancy had been problem-free. Several months later, I saw her again, along with her little boy who had grown much calmer. She told me that, since last seeing me, she had remembered the following event: "When I was six months pregnant, I saw the assassination of President Sadat live on television. It really shocked me, and for the rest of the pregnancy my baby moved around so much that when he was born the umbilical cord was wrapped around his neck several times!"

A pregnant woman who experiences a very strong fright can, in severe cases, go into premature labor. The scenario is fairly common—a six-month-pregnant woman is rushed to the hospital already dilated and everyone fears the worst. In such cases, when the fundamental issue for the child is "To be or not to be?" the indicated remedy is **Opium** because the endorphins—the opiates secreted by our brain—control fear, pain, respiration, and other vital functions such as digestion.

In other cases, a baby may be born underweight, hypersomniac, constipated, or a poor feeder. It may even stop breathing in its sleep, leading to Sudden Infant Death Syndrome. A dose of Opium will help to restore order and prevent the worst in such cases.

One young woman I saw had been hospitalized for threatened miscarriage in her sixth month of pregnancy. She had gone into shock after watching a group of skiers try to escape from an avalanche. Her son subsequently presented with deep-seated anxieties, which were cured with a few doses of Opium.

**Staphysagria** is the remedy for frustration, as well as for abusive, sadomasochistic situations—such as those experienced by women whose employers are so furious at them for "falling" pregnant that they punish them with the most strenuous jobs. These are hypersensitive women who don't enjoy being pregnant. They are especially averse to the medical check-ups, which involve having to undress and expose their private parts to staff who are frequently lacking in tact. Each vaginal examination is experienced as a rape and reminds them of that first, highly painful sexual experience which left them with a classic bout of "honeymoon cystitis."

All this suppressed anger and indignation is expressed by the baby during its first three months, in the form of colic. The baby sleeps during the day but cries all night and goes on to become the kind of child who "asks for punishment" by placing himself in abusive situations—until the day he receives Staphysagria. His mother will say, "Please give me a remedy—this child is pushing me to the limit and I'm scared of really hurting him one day."

For the pregnant woman, the forthcoming labor is often a major source of anxiety. She loses sleep, wondering whether she will survive the birth and if the baby will be normal, and the fetus starts to becomes agitated. A dose of **Actea Racemosa** will restore her confidence and equilibrium and even enable her to avoid the Biblical curse of painful labor.

**Pulsatilla** is the remedy for fear of separation. Mother and child are so happily absorbed in their all-consuming love for each other that they will do anything to put off the inevitable. The baby malpositions itself, the mother fails to go into labor at the right time. Homeopaths in India routinely give a dose of Pulsatilla 15C towards the end of pregnancy, to encourage correct presentation of the baby and a problem-free labor.

**Sepia** is for those who feel torn between the role of being a mother and that of being a woman. They experience pregnancy as a loss of their femininity and unconsciously reject the child. The first three months of gestation are marked by nausea and frequent vomiting, followed by the development of chloasma (the "mask of pregnancy"). The last few months are ruined by constipation and lower back pains.

**Symphoricarpus racemosa** is the remedy for very serious vomiting, which is so profuse that it endangers the lives of both mother and baby. Such symptoms represent an unconscious attempt to abort the child via the mouth.

**Apis** is another remedy for threatened miscarriage in the third month. This is the stage at which the embryo becomes a fetus, with all the vital organs now in place. Apis, the crushed bee, is a major allergy remedy. In these cases, the unborn baby is perceived by the mother's body as an allergen, which it needs to get rid of. Apis rejects the other person and the idea of belonging to a family or community, like that of the bee in its hive.

Finally, we mustn't forget the stresses caused by certain modern medical procedures such as ultrasound—a technique that has proved invaluable for identifying potentially problematic labors and serious fetal abnormalities. However, when the mother's gynecologist tells her she is expecting twins, for example, she finds herself plunged into a state of duality. She wonders which of the two babies she will love, and the bond between mother and child is damaged. The trauma of such an experience remains even if, as sometimes happens at the next examination, the doctor can only find one baby. Cases such as this need **Anacardium orientalis**—the remedy of impossible choices.

Without a dose of Anacardium, these children will go on to have terrible problems making decisions—whether to act childishly or grown-up; whether to be good or naughty. One moment they're lovely and cuddly, the next horribly rude. They are constantly having to decide whether to side with the angel on one shoulder or the devil on the other. Adolescence is especially difficult for them and at school they find it impossible to decide which subjects to study and which career to pursue.

Amniocentesis is undoubtedly one of the most stressful medical procedures. When the doctor arrives with a huge needle to pierce the womb and extract some of its amniotic fluid, the baby retreats into a corner and the mother becomes extremely tense, as she is unconsciously reminded of the old abortion needles.

I once received a call from a panic-stricken mother who had been taken to the hospital. The amniocentesis test had gone wrong, her waters were leaking, and she'd been told she would lose the baby. The first remedy prescribed was Opium 15C, for the fear which was disrupting her energy state, then several hours later a dose of Silica 15C—which enabled her to bring the pregnancy to term.

**Silica** is the remedy for those who can't and won't come out of their shell and who panic if they have to speak in public. They are hypersensitive people who tend to hide their brilliance and remain in the background. When they do manage to overcome their anxiety, they surprise everyone with their flashes of genius. They have an extreme fear of sharp objects and especially of injections, which makes them easy to spot on vaccination day! When stressed, they sweat profusely and very offensively from the hands and feet.

In addition, Silica has the delusion that it "does not own its left side." As we have seen, the left side represents the world of feelings, which Silica suppresses deep within for fear of exposing his true self to others.

**Ignatia** is the remedy for children who were deprived for several days (which seem like centuries to the unborn baby) of their mother's love, while the latter awaited the results of amniocentesis and emotionally detached themselves from their baby in case they would have to abort. These children are extremely sensitive to broken relationships, which make them withdraw into themselves with lots of weeping, sighing, and somatised symptoms such as sore throats, coughs and the "lump in the throat."

**Aurum metallicum** is the remedy for women who have lots of abortions, as noted by Kent in his *Materia Medica*. Aurums see themselves as the Sun, as God—at the center of everything and with a corresponding power over life and death. They rashly defy the laws of nature, until one day their sense of guilt drives them into a state of suicidal despair.

## PRIMUM NON NOCERE

Hippocrates told his followers "First, do no harm." Good things always come in moderation, so doctors must resist the temptation to over-prescribe for pregnant women—especially since the majority of allopathic medicines are contra-indicated during pregnancy. Some antibiotics will damage the baby's hearing, while others will stain its teeth.

We should also guard against untimely doses of fluoride "to strengthen the teeth." We've all heard the saying "A baby, a tooth" and it is understandable for a young woman to want to protect her teeth with careful cleaning. But we should avoid making the mental leap from there to an overloading of both mother and unborn baby with fluoride. This can create a "fluoric taint," producing congenital abnormalities such as webbed feet, misshapen ears, extra fingers, twin ureters, and cleft lips and palates. By the same token, a dose of **Calcarea fluorica** 15C at the start of pregnancy will prevent the development of a cleft lip or palate.

There are of course many other toxic substances that pregnant women should avoid. In first place comes tobacco, which produces stunted children due to poor oxygenation of the fetus and atrophy of the placenta. **Tabacum** should always be considered as a possible remedy for any under-developed child whose parents are smokers.

Second comes alcohol, which produces puny, hyperactive children who require a dose of **(Ethyl) Alcohol.** And finally, there are all the modern-day street drugs—cannabis, cocaine, and heroine—all of which create energetic blocks which will need to be cleared (with **Cannabis indica, Coca** and **Opium** respectively) for the child to develop properly.

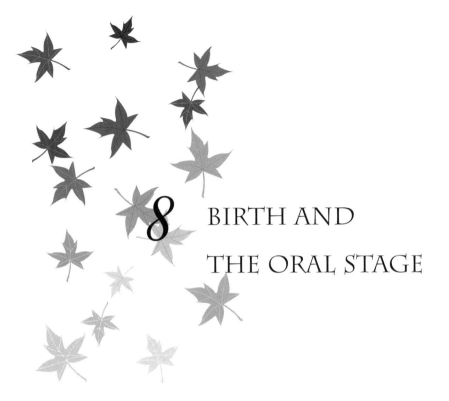

# 8 BIRTH AND THE ORAL STAGE

Birth is the most vital step in life—literally, the first move!

We go through a tunnel and emerge into a bright light—it all sounds strangely similar to the experiences of people who have had Near Death Experiences (the final move!). But in this case, it isn't unconditional love, truth, and warmth that greet us, but the fluorescent lights of a room that more often than not resembles an operating theatre. Thanks to the epidural, Mom can't feel anything, and the resulting weakness of her contractions often means that forceps have to be used to pull the head out.

In natural circumstances, the baby has to want to be born since it is the one who sets the whole process in motion by releasing certain hormones. Nowadays, however, it is often the gynecologist who decides to induce birth at a time convenient for him, through the administration of oxytocin, for example. It is interesting to note how few babies are born on Christmas Day or January 1st!

Babies who have been induced in this way will often register their displeasure with a chronic gastric reflux. This is where the peristaltic motions of the esophagus continue to move from the stomach up towards the mouth, just like in the womb when they enabled the baby to regurgitate amniotic fluid. The babies refuse to change to the mouth-stomach direction, necessary if food is to be digested correctly. This causes numerous problems, since the highly acidic gastric juices may enter the upper respiratory tract, leading to nasopharyngitis and otitis, or even the lower tract, causing bronchitis or sudden death in the event of a particularly copious reflux.

**Asafoetida** can be an effective cure for gastric reflux and is especially indicated in cases where the mother had slight mastitis with milk secretion at the birth (this latter symptom may also indicate **Cyclamen** or **Tuberculinum**).

Chloe was a lovely little eight-year-old girl who had been prone to violent attacks of asthma since the age of two. These attacks were so severe that she sometimes needed to be hospitalized and was taking a lot of allopathic drugs, including cortisone. Various homeopathic remedies had been tried, without success.

One day, I observed her having an attack and what struck me most of all was her constant whining and her refusal to be carried or even consoled. This suggested **Cina,** a well-known remedy for worms. On asking the mother, I was informed that the girl received worming treatment three times a year. Cina is also a remedy for encephalitis following a lumbar puncture, and when I mentioned this, the mother told me she had fainted during labor when she was given an epidural, and the baby had been subjected to an emergency delivery by forceps. I asked her if she had ever received a lumbar puncture before then, and she told me that when she was seven she contracted meningitis which was treated in the hospital. Since receiving a dose of Cina, Chloe has had no more asthma attacks.

Even when the labor goes well and there isn't too much intervention, the baby still experiences a fear of abandonment on leaving his warm, loving environment and finding himself naked and exposed to the cold.

Aurélie came to see me about her baby's history of recurrent bronchitis. When I asked her why she thought her child was ill, she said, "I'll tell you something I told my first doctor, but he laughed at me. Immediately after my daughter was born, the midwife bathed her in water that I thought was too cold. Even in the maternity hospital, Aurélie already had a cold and she's never been well since."

**Antimonium crudum** is the main remedy for symptoms following a cold bath or shower, or any sudden break in the warmth of maternal love. Afterwards, the child can't stand to be touched or even watched and tends to be extremely ticklish.

## THE BREATH OF LIFE

If we don't start breathing within three minutes of birth, we die. Once the umbilical cord has been cut, oxygen stops flowing into us from our mother, and carbon dioxide begins to accumulate in the body. When the $CO_2$ reaches a certain level, respiration is triggered by specific areas of the brain. This is our first major step, the first life sequence: Carbon dioxide = Respiration = Joy of being alive.

Smokers go through the same sequence when they light a cigarette every time they have to face any ordeal or take some major or minor step in life. This even extends to the last cigarette of the condemned man!

The source of most respiratory diseases is to be found at this moment of the first breath. An asthmatic, for example, can take oxygen in but can't then expel it, so his lungs remain filled with stale air. Inspiration must be followed by expiration—we must give in order to receive a fresh supply of oxygen. This refusal to give symbolizes a refusal to live outside the womb and a desire to stay inside the mother, where we are protected from allergens, the environment, and other people. Someone who goes into acute respiratory failure may have to be put on a ventilator, a system that mimics that of blood oxygenation via the placenta.

## THE BREAD OF LIFE

Having mastered the art of breathing, we go on to the second of life's sequences: Hunger = Food = Pleasure. Since we have now stopped receiving glucose via the umbilical cord, our blood sugar levels start to drop and we are once again faced with the prospect of death and start to cry. Fortunately, the mother is there with her colostrum (the first milk, which is rich in sugars and antibodies) or with a bottle, if she is unable to feed.

The reason that smokers who try to give up often put on weight is that they are once again having to pass through this second sequence of life.

## THE WARMTH OF LIFE

Finally, there is the joy of being warmed and caressed by the mother and it is at this point that many skin diseases such as psoriasis and eczema begin. Eczema, for example, is a somatization of the child's mourning for its very first protective layer of the womb, and of its subsequent reluctance to break through the skin of its cocoon-like relationship with the mother.

One day, a mother brought me her seventeen-year-old daughter who had been covered with eczema since the age of eighteen months. Coming from a medical family, the two women had already consulted the best practitioners in their area but without success.

Looking at the girl, the thought came to me that she was beautiful but untouchable. It transpired that when she was eighteen months of age, her mother decided to leave her with her grandmother for a week, while she attended a conference in the USA. Unfortunately, on the day of her departure, the grandmother fell ill and the child had to be hurriedly entrusted to an aunt who she didn't know. By the time her parents returned, the little girl was covered in eczema.

I explained to the girl that her skin problems were caused by her refusal to break the physical bond with her mother, but that at the age of seventeen, her caresses should be reserved for someone other than her mother! Three days later, not a single trace of the eczema remained.


## PROBLEM BIRTHS

Sometimes, the process of birth goes wrong and produces physical trauma. The baby emerges looking like it's just done ten rounds in the boxing ring, with its face all swollen and distorted. (Perhaps the popularity of boxing as a sport is due to people's unconscious memories of their passage into the outside world?)

**Arnica** is the first remedy to give for these initial traumas— these first "blows of life." Without it, these patients will become masochists who get a kick out of working themselves to death. They refuse to delegate and metaphorically beat themselves up, until it finally becomes too much for them and they collapse. They are like the first marathon runner, who ran all the way to Athens to announce the Greeks' victory over Persia, but then immediately died from an overstrained heart.

**Hypericum** is the remedy for trauma caused by forceps and traction of the spinal cord, as well as for nerves that have been damaged or stretched during the baby's passage along the birth canal. These are children who may go on to develop eczema on the face, asthma that is aggravated by foggy weather, or tetanus. Hypericum is also the remedy for dislocation of the coccyx in the mother following labor. The sacrum derives its name from the Latin *os sacrum* or "holy bone," since it was once used in sacrifices. The baby therefore receives the holy sacrament by passing over the mother's sacrum in its descent towards the light.

**Aconite** is the remedy for emergency situations and especially hemorrhaging of the mother that starts around 11:00 P.M. This may be caused by a potentially fatal condition such as placenta praevia, where the placenta is implanted near or over the opening to the cervix. This is a potentially fatal condition that needs to be handled with care and expertise in order to avoid long-term damage or death of both the mother and her baby. Children who survive such a traumatic birth but haven't yet received a dose of Aconite are never "a bit poorly." When they fall ill (usually around midnight or midday) it is always with an urgent and life-threatening condition such as croupous laryngitis, where the baby suddenly starts to choke and emits a harsh, barking cough.

**Carbo vegetabilis,** or vegetable charcoal, is made by heating organic matter in the absence of air, and will only burn if it is reoxygenated. It is the remedy for blue babies—children who do not start to breathe straight away and who have to be stimulated, oxygenated, and have their airways cleared. They have a low score on the Apgar scale—the system that records the infant's heart rate, respiration, and response rate one minute after birth.

These are children who have difficulty developing normally and who fail to recover fully from childhood diseases such as whooping cough and measles. Apart from the fact that they need lots of fresh air and want to be fanned constantly, these patients are instantly recognizable by their marbled skin, thread-veined cheeks, and, during adolescence, acne-covered back. They have a craving for tobacco, since cigarettes contain their remedy in material doses. However, smoking gradually aggravates their condition, leading eventually to respiratory insufficiency.

**Argentum nitricum** has a special significance at birth, since medical staff have been dropping silver nitrate into the eyes of newborns as a prophylactic against ophthalmia for many years. This mixture of silver—the material substance—and volatile nitric acid, is a potent symbol of the spirit's painful incarnation into matter. The baby cries at birth because he knows he has entered a world where space and time are perceived as finite. This spatio-temporal finiteness is torture to Argentum nitricum, who breaks down if he has a deadline to meet or finds himself in a confined space. These are nervous, hurried people who are constantly running around as though their lives depended on it, since "Time is money" (and both are finite!). They have forgotten that they also belong to another world, in which time and space are infinite, and so they are often atheists.

Argentum nitricums who can overcome their fear of heights may indulge in sports such as parachuting or the high-dive, which involve throwing themselves into the void and thereby reliving that initial fall to Earth.

**Causticum** tends to have a difficult birth. The shoulders won't come through and the baby ends up with a fractured clavicle or even paralysis of the brachial plexus—the network of spinal nerves that supply the upper limbs. Later, they will have a constant fear of impending disaster—like Damocles, they are waiting for the sword to fall on them and fracture their clavicle again. They use their physical fragility to manipulate everyone around them, saying things like "I'm so weak, could you do this for me?" and sympathize with others because "But for the grace of God ..." They may go on to suffer from convulsions followed by paralysis.

**Opium** is the remedy for the ultimate trauma—cardio-respiratory failure. It is invaluable for sluggish, constipated babies who feed poorly, especially if there is an umbilical hernia. Such children are prone to relapse and, in severe cases, sudden death.

**Natrum sulphuricum** has had a knock on the head, causing cerebral edema. There is too much water—too much humor (from the Latin *humor*, "fluid")—in the brain, and it is literally the baby's humor that suffers. Each time he's hungry and isn't fed immediately, he goes into a profound depression that changes to overexcitement when the milk finally arrives. Such marked alternation between extreme sadness and excessive joy can result in a lifelong manic-depressive disorder. These patients often suffer from asthma in wet weather and develop oozing warts.

Finally, **Kali carbonicum** can't tolerate its own dependency during the first few months of life. When we don't eat regularly, the resulting drop in blood sugar cuts off the supply of energy to the sodium pump—the biological system that maintains a high concentration of potassium within the cells and a high concentration of sodium outside. The baby screams and cries until his mother arrives and feeds him. Immediately afterwards, she is angrily rejected by a child who is furious with his own dependency. These babies go on to become children who desire other people's company but then treat them outrageously. They crave sugar and often go into asthma attacks at around 3 A.M., with a concomitant stitching pain in the chest. They are often dyslexic, with the specific symptom that they confuse the "m" and the "n." Later on, they will place themselves in situations of dependency (with drugs, for example) and see everything in terms of black and white.

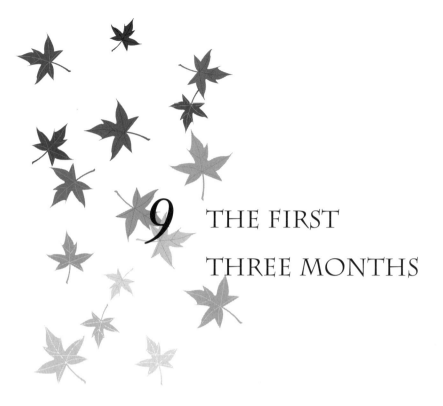

# 9 THE FIRST THREE MONTHS

Adapting to life outside the womb isn't always an easy process and can create problems. All attention is focused on the baby's growth, which is extremely rapid and often leads to an overloading of the digestive system. This manifests as colic, gas, and flatulence, even when the baby is receiving only its mother's milk which is specifically adapted to its needs. Mothers should beware of taking too many vitamins, since these will produce a highly-strung baby, while taking fluoride "to strengthen the teeth" often results in a blocked nose. A blocked nose will eventually become permanent due to enlargement of the adenoids, followed by recurrent bouts of otitis that leave tell-tale calcium deposits on the eardrums.

**Calcarea fluorica** is the specific remedy for such symptoms, as well as for obstruction of the lachrymal glands. Other remedies to think of include **Argentum nitricum, Calcarea carbonica,**

**Natrum muriaticum, Pulsatilla,** and **Silica.**

**Nux vomica** is the best remedy for an overworked digestive system, where the child is overloaded with vitamins and totally stressed out by its hectic existence. This is another remedy that will unblock the nose and enable the baby to sleep at night.

Children suffering from severe attacks of colic may need **Cuprum Metallicum** if their swallowing is accompanied by gurgling sounds, or **Colocynthis** if they go into violent temper tantrums and have to bend double.

Cuprum is one of the first remedies to think of if the child goes into convulsions, and it can be especially miraculous in cases of West syndrome—a kind of encephalitis that deforms the brain. Cuprum's underlying theme is "I feel like this situation is above my head. I'm not up to it." It is significant that in many parts of the world, copper is put on plants to protect them during their growth period.

Excessive sweating from the head that results in the gradual formation of cradle cap is an indication for **Calcarea carbonica.** This remedy is ideal for children who put on weight rapidly and who are extremely fearful, with the cradle cap being an attempt to protect their delicate fontanelles. Calcarea carbonica is acutely conscious of the vulnerability of the human body—protected as it is only by the skeleton—and tries to make up for this by feeding greedily and layering on fat.

Other children are the opposite and refuse to eat. This is the case with **Silica,** which even rejects his mother's breast. He has problems adapting to life outside the womb and loves hot baths, which remind him of the joy he experienced before birth.

**Lycopodium** would like to gobble up not only the breast but the mother herself, in order to enjoy absolute power. He suffers from wind and abdominal bloating and goes into violent temper tantrums. He experiences red, sandy deposits in his urine (uric acid). He will later be prone to gout.

The Lycopodium child is obsessed with growing up, because to be grown-up means to have power. Mothers of Lycopodium babies often find that milk flows from the right breast only. In such cases, it is the mother who should be given the remedy.

**Lachesis** is the antithesis of Lycopodium, being indicated when only the left breast produces milk. Babies needing Lachesis often narrowly escaped death when they were born because the umbilical cord was wrapped around their neck. Other symptoms of Lachesis include thread-veined cheeks and an umbilical hernia.

**Aethusa cynapium** suffers from a communication breakdown between mother and child. Every time the baby cries in order to express something, its mother doesn't know what to do and, hoping for the best, feeds it. Gorged with milk, the baby throws it all up and two hours later starts to cry again. These are children who will go on to have a milk allergy.

By the time it is one month old, a baby is able to recognize faces and smile at them. At three months, it can hold up its head and see someone on the other side of the room. From three to six months, the baby usually goes through a quiet stage where it is happy just to be alive. It feeds regularly, four times a day, and sleeps peacefully.

## VACCINATIONS

Parents should avoid over-vaccinating their baby during the first few months in an attempt to protect it from every possible illness. Vaccination is often seen as a kind of insurance against fatal disease. But if we spend all our money on insurance, there is none left to buy food and so we still die. It is like describing life itself as a sexually-transmitted and inevitably fatal disease!

People are pressurized into having too many vaccinations these days. In some countries, it is not unusual for a child to receive nineteen inoculations by the age of four months — three lots of Hepatitis B, a BCG, plus three doses of a DPT/hemophilia/whooping cough combination!

Such excesses need to stop, because the immune disorders they produce are creating a generation of asthmatics. Asthma, with its impeded respiration and congested lungs, tends to be blamed on environmental pollution and exposure to cigarette smoke but is more usually triggered by these first inoculations.

Some people refuse all vaccinations, which I believe to be unreasonable. Among these abstainers, some put their trust in organic foods and a healthy lifestyle. This is the case with **Calcarea silica** who, as we've already seen, often remains attached to people who have long been dead—telling them their problems and asking their advice. Others abstain after seeing a family member fall seriously ill after a vaccination, a situation that brings to mind **Thuja, Silica,** or **Sulphur.**

Some people are the opposite and want every vaccine available. **Arsenicum album,** for instance, wants to protect himself from death at any price!

I believe early vaccination to be pointless, since up to the age of nine months the baby is protected by antibodies received via the mother's placenta before birth (while the antibodies received in breast milk protect the digestive tract against gastro-enteritis).

The whooping cough vaccine carries many risks (such as encephalitis) and can cause asthma, so should be reserved for children who are already socializing. I believe two injections to be more than enough to protect a child for the first year of life—the only time when whooping cough poses any threat. However, the whooping cough vaccination should be avoided altogether when the child has a family history of epilepsy or asthma or had a difficult birth. In cases of persistent cough following vaccination, the first remedy to give is **Carbo vegetabilis** 30C, which should redress the balance.

As for BCG, while its efficacy remains unproven, it is a well-known trigger for asthma and allergies. Following the BCG vaccination, **Silica** develops a suppurating wound that refuses to heal. Since the pus produced contains live tuberculous bacteria, everyone he comes into contact with is at risk of contamination—especially people suffering from immune disorders such as AIDS and people on immuno-suppressant drugs or cortisone treatment. Such patients should be treated locally with an anti-tubercular and antibiotic ointment, as well as internally with doses of **Silica** (15 to 30C) and **Tuberculinum** (15 to 30C).

Finally, should children be vaccinated against measles, rubella, and mumps? First of all, it seems totally unnatural to put three such unrelated viruses together in a single vaccine. Secondly, the vaccine does not protect for as long as the disease itself. And thirdly, the fragility of these vaccines means that they are easily destroyed, by exposure to heat for example. In other words, we run the risk of creating epidemics of measles, mumps, and rubella among the adult population, who are much less able to tolerate such diseases. What's more, the eradication by vaccines of childhood diseases most likely affects and changes the immune system. This is a problem that affects the whole of society and should therefore be debated much more thoroughly than it has been to date.

In my opinion, all other vaccinations are superfluous—meningitis, for example, being rare in many parts of the world and usually reserved for children living in large groups. As for Hepatitis B, in two decades of pediatric practice in France, I haven't seen a single case in a child under fourteen. What's more, this genetically-produced vaccine does not yet carry a reliable guarantee of safety and has been linked to numerous serious side-effects such as multiple sclerosis, sight problems, various auto-immune diseases, and diabetes.

## GUARDIANSHIP

Guardianship of the child is a real problem in modern societies where, despite the high rate of unemployment, pregnant women and young mothers usually have no option but to continue working. This runs directly contrary to the findings of Freud, which demonstrated the importance of the mother-child bond during the first year of life.

Children who are placed in nurseries and group situations too early often suffer from feelings of abandonment and disorientation. The **Capsicum** child, for instance, becomes prone to repeated bouts of glue ear and seeks refuge in food to the extent that he may become seriously overweight.

Other children may on the contrary feel quite at home in such a group setting. This is the case with **Sulphur,** who immediately adapts to all sorts of situations and is very gregarious. The mother is often happy to leave him, since she feels fulfilled by her own work outside the house.

Sometimes it is the grandmother who looks after the child, in which case everyone involved should take care to ensure that she doesn't literally take the mother's place and deprive the latter of her own child. Grandparents need to play a different, more lenient role than the parents. Otherwise, the child may become confused, leading to possible psychological conflicts in later life.

Future societies will one day understand the need for parental leave lasting at least two years—the first year to be spent with the mother, the second with either the mother or the father. The temporary job vacancies created will be filled by people on the unemployment register, and young babies will once again be allowed to develop in a normal environment. Children will not be sent to nursery or a babysitter until the end of the oral stage (between eighteen and twenty-four months).


## PACIFIERS

The pacifier is a sort of masturbation of the oral stage. By sucking, the baby remains in a state of constant pleasure but runs the danger of cutting himself off from the outside world. If insomnia sets in, it is because the baby falls asleep while still sucking—just as though at his mother's breast—and wakes briefly but frequently throughout the night. Each time he awakes, the baby looks and cries for his mother and the whole situation becomes intolerable. The only solution in such cases is to throw away the pacifier and give a support such as **Pulsatilla.** This is the archetypal remedy for a baby who doesn't want to leave its mother and who falls asleep in her arms. Or is it the mother who doesn't want to leave her baby? If in doubt, give the remedy to both!

**Arsenicum album,** the remedy for fear of death, is top of the list for insomnia problems, since sleep is experienced as a "little death"—the body rests while the soul goes wandering and only returns the next morning when we awake. The mothers of children needing Arsenicum have often been severely affected by a death, sometimes even during the pregnancy. The baby is agitated and "lively," and doesn't sleep between midnight and 3:00 A.M.

**Medorrhinum** is for babies who can only get to sleep crouched on their front like a little frog, and who often develop diaper rash. Since the mother has been told to lay her baby on its back in order to avoid the risk of Sudden Infant Death Syndrome, the result is chronic insomnia. Medorrhinum is also unable to sleep in high-altitude places, but is better near the sea.

Other remedies to think of are **Staphysagria,** which sleeps all day and cries all night; **Capsicum,** which can't sleep when away from home; and **Ignatia,** whose insomnia is due to a love disappointment experienced in the womb (the break-up of the parents, for example) or else an amniocentesis test which has disturbed its equilibrium.

**Carcinosin** is the remedy for babies who have never slept through the night. The child often has a lot of birthmarks or *café au lait* marks and has a bluish tinge to the sclera. It is the remedy for people who have never managed to break the bond with their mother.

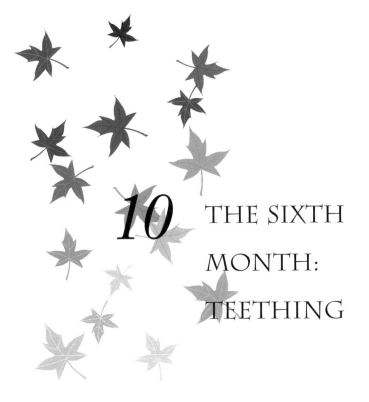

# 10 THE SIXTH MONTH: TEETHING

The sixth month of life usually coincides with teething. The very act of teething can provoke illness, because the piercing of the gums creates pain and inflammation which can extend to the pharynx, ears (otitis), and respiratory tract. Theoreticians claim such illnesses are caused by germs and viruses. They are right up to a point, but it is above all poverty of the soil and resulting imbalances in the bacterial or viral flora that are to blame for any problems provoked by teething.

The cutting of the first milk tooth symbolizes the first step towards adulthood, because it is thanks to our teeth that we are able to eat and be weaned, and therefore to become independent from the mother. Any problems caused by the emergence of our first teeth reflect those created by our emergence from the womb— our initial separation from the mother—and it is mostly the same homeopathic remedies that apply.

**Chamomilla,** for example, is for pain that is so unbearable and seems so unfair that it makes the child very angry and restless. This remedy is characterized by the fact that one cheek is very red and hot while the other is pale. The child is better when being held and rocked and when traveling in a car.

**Rhus toxicodendron** is the remedy for sore throats and respiratory problems caused by teething. The fever usually comes on in the middle of the night, between 1 A.M. and 3:00 A.M., and the child is restless and very chilly, with pains all over the body. The tongue is particularly characteristic—white with a red tip.

**Phytolacca** presents with pains that radiate to the ears and a constant need to bite on something hard.

**Podophyllum** suffers from profuse, gushing, yellowish diarrhea and sometimes develops a rectal prolapse.

The stools of **Rheum palmatum** are so acidic and sour that they can be smelled from the other side of the room.

**Calcarea bromata** becomes sleepless when teething. He doesn't feel safe in his own home, despite being surrounded by his family.

**Magnesia muriatica** suffers from constipation during teething, with small round stools like sheep's dung. This remedy is often indicated in babies born to parents who have gone against the tide by moving back to nature and away from the violence of city life.

Once the baby's teeth have developed, it is able to bite—a gesture it uses to express itself, gain independence from its mother's breast, and affirm its identity for the first time. The adult within the child starts to emerge and prepares to "get its teeth into" life. But they also become aware that life can be a question of "eat or be eaten" and that they are caught between the "jaws of death," which provokes a fear of dying. Their dreams become filled with devouring monsters—wolves, sharks, and dinosaurs.

**Stramonium** is particularly prone to such night terrors. He wakes up screaming and doesn't recognize his parents, who have difficulty calming him down.

**Belladonna** screams at the approach of a stranger. He goes into a state of feverish delirium around 8:00 P.M., with a hot, red skin and dilated pupils, and sees visions of hideous faces.

One of my patient's babies hadn't slept a wink, ever since his mother had broken her nose in a car accident and ended up with a huge, disfiguring bandage over the middle of her face. The baby would start screaming as soon as anyone came near and smiled at him, and he was prone to violent nightmares before midnight. The situation was quickly rectified by a dose of Belladonna 30C.

This oral stage is often resolved by one of the childhood diseases such as measles, German measles, or mumps—all of which act as a rite of passage to the next stage of development. My own daughter had a severe bout of measles around the age of eighteen months. Her temperature went over 104 degrees, her eyes started to suppurate, and she became delirious. The fact that her lower limbs were cold enabled me to prescribe Stramonium, which cured her very rapidly. All this happened shortly after an incident in which her mother, who was six months pregnant, had had to watch helplessly as the postman was attacked by our wolf-dog.

Interestingly enough, it is often the emergence of the child's canine teeth that poses the most problems. Canine comes from the Latin *canis* ("the dog"), with *canis lupus* meaning "wolf." The very purpose of childhood diseases is to strengthen the immune system and guard against disorders such as lupus.

Measles, which is caused by the *morbillinum* virus, killed many children in primitive societies, where it was common for mothers to have a child every eighteen months throughout their fertile period. When a child died from this disease, it was due to not having spent enough time in the fusional bond of the oral stage before having to make way for its new sibling. Absolutely devastated by this sudden rupture with the mother, they would fall ill and die, thereby ensuring that only the very strongest children survived—three per couple, on average.

Fearful **Calcarea carbonica** is terrified by the level of aggression associated with the oral stage of development. His dentition is slow and difficult, and he will later be afraid of animals—especially dogs—since this is the constitutional of Belladonna.

**Silica** prefers not to teethe at all! At worst, he produces a dental inclusion, where the tooth is unable to erupt because of excessive surrounding tissue—just like the person he may become, preferring to spend the rest of his life withdrawn into his shell. Only a sharp object can pierce the shell, which is the very thing he fears most. Silica is well-known for its ability to expulse foreign bodies, and is also the best remedy for very delayed dentition (after the twelfth month for the first tooth).

**Drosera** is a carnivorous plant that devours any insect that lands on its leaves. It is a good remedy for coughs, teething, whooping cough, and tuberculosis.

Tuberculosis is the disease of people who would rather leave their bodies than live in this cruel, hostile world. Simone Weil, the French mystic who died of TB in 1939, spoke of her "voluntary self-destruction in order to fuse with God." **Tuberculinum** doesn't usually go so far, but does dream of traveling, of distant lands, of paradise, and the grandeur of snow-topped mountain peaks.

**Hydrophobinum,** which is prepared from the rabies virus, has the most extreme fear of being devoured. Hydrophobinum children are constantly biting and want to control everything. They can't bear bright lights, are afraid of water (like Cannabis indica), and love chocolate. They have commonly been bitten by a dog at some point and grow up into highly intrusive adults who desire complete control over their friends and family.

Every time he cuts a tooth, **Kreosotum** comes down with a bad cough, and sometimes even bronchiolitis with respiratory distress. One characteristic physical symptom is diaper rash with every new tooth, with red-raw buttocks. The teeth themselves are fragile and decay rapidly. It is as though Kreosotum refuses to accept the aggression symbolized by his new teeth, preferring instead to have them eaten away and destroyed. Later on, as teenagers and adults, they are subject to dreams of rape, and there is often a history of incest or rape in the family—in other words, of violent penetration. Kreosotum's reaction is to reject all forms of aggression, making life impossible.

Kreosote is beech wood tar, the smoke of which is used to preserve meat and animal flesh. But for life to be preserved, it is *spirit* that must penetrate the flesh.

The oral stage leaves its mark on society, as demonstrated by the success of such movies as *Jurassic Park* and *Jaws*. Animals bare their teeth as a warning that they are about to attack, while humans are the opposite—we bare our teeth as an act of love, in order to smile. The whole of humanity is defined by this opposite behavior, and it is by the quality of a person's smile that we recognize true love.

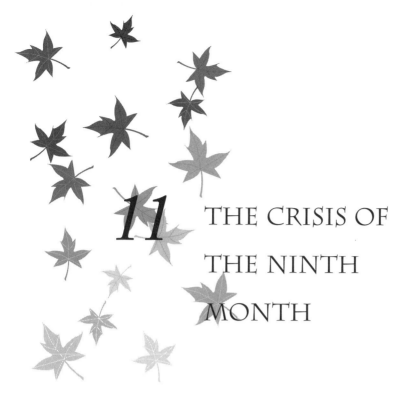

# 11  THE CRISIS OF THE NINTH MONTH

The ninth month of life brings with it memories of the ninth and final month of gestation, and of birth. The baby goes into a state of separation anxiety and doesn't want to leave its parents.

At around twelve months, the baby starts to walk and even if disabled should be encouraged and enabled to stand upright. Here again, the human path diverges from that of the animal, with the arms and hands being freed for work and creativity. It is this that has enabled us to develop intelligence and brain capacity.

Learning to walk brings its falls, bangs, and bumps, but in the end it always works out well and gives us undreamt-of independence. It is at this time that parents must take extra care not to leave objects within reach, and to keep the child away from toxic substances and other potential dangers such as power outlets and cookers!

Many people wonder about the benefits of babywalkers, which enable the still crawling child to move around the house. On the one hand, these may delay the development of proper walking, with the baby frightened to let go of its support. On the other hand, he may benefit greatly from this early taste of independence and autonomy.

Even without a babywalker, the child can get around on all fours and start exploring its environment. As it becomes more mobile, it is gradually able to widen its field of discovery to take in more and more of the world outside.

From eleven to eighteen months, the baby returns to a state of relative calm and stability, leaving it free to develop the necessary motor skills and speech. It is important to monitor the development of the major senses of vision (warning bells should sound if the child starts to squint or bumps into doors) and hearing, which may be impeded by recurrent bouts of otitis.

**Tuberculinium Aviaire,** Chicken Tuberculosis, is the main remedy for recurrent otitis in newborns. It will restore order in tubercular children—those who react badly to the BCG, are worse at the seaside, and better in the mountains. They often have white marks on their nails and a visible vein at the root of the nose.

**Cyclamen** is an excellent remedy for childhood strabismus, especially where the left eye turns inwards. The mother often has a secret sorrow (the child's father is not the man she loved, for example), but she can't talk about it and ridicules everything.

**Cicuta virosa** is a remedy for strabismus following a bang on the head, such as that caused by a fall or post-natal trauma. The child fails to develop and progress, preferring to remain a baby since to him the adult world seems insane.

In cases of strabismus, it is important to check for amblyopia— a reduction or dimness of vision due to only one eye functioning properly while the other atrophies. The good eye should be covered in order to make the lazy one work harder. Otherwise, the child risks losing its sight in the one eye and being forced to see the world in two dimensions.

## CHILDREN WHO DON'T WALK

Sometimes, a child doesn't start to walk until very late—sixteen months or even later—despite the absence of any neurological disability. Homeopathy can help in such instances.

**Calcarea carbonica** is for fearful children who have poor muscle tone and are often overweight.

**Causticum** also lacks the necessary muscle tone.

**Sulphur** doesn't want to make any effort. He couldn't care less about walking and is quite happy to remain in his lazy state of bliss.

**Baryta carbonica** doesn't understand how much joy he'll get from walking.

**Agaricus** is awkward and clumsy.

**Natrum muriaticum** doesn't want to leave its mother in order to follow the father, while **Silica** is unnerved by strangers and refuses to go towards them.

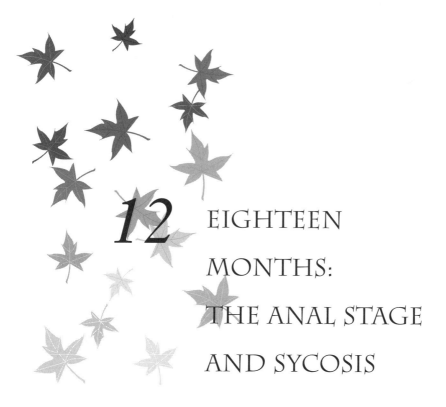

# 12 EIGHTEEN MONTHS: THE ANAL STAGE AND SYCOSIS

The eighteenth month of life signals the end of the oral stage and of the fusional bond with the mother, which started to loosen around nine months. The father plays an increasingly important role as the child passes into the anal stage. The baby starts to gain control of its sphincters and use the potty, enabling it to keep its diaper clean. It is at this time that the baby's bottle and pacifier should also be abandoned, since these objects will only serve to prolong the oral stage and delay the natural progression out of diapers. The child must leave the old behind—otherwise his poor parents will be condemned to many more months of diaper-changing!

The **Pulsatilla** child refuses to break his fusional bond with the mother, along with everything it represents. He takes his bottle and teddy bear everywhere with him, with the latter serving as a symbol for the placenta that linked him to his mother.

I had one young patient who never went anywhere without

his blue rabbit. This toy was totally real for him, to the extent that when he went sailing with his parents one day and his father told him to be careful not to drop his rabbit in the sea, he instantly replied, "Yes, because there are no carrots in the sea!" He suffered from severe eczema, which rapidly disappeared with repeated doses of Pulsatilla 7C.

Other signs pointing to Pulsatilla are warm-bloodedness and a lack of thirst (except for sugared water from his bottle). He may appear reckless and will happily jump into a swimming pool or lake, but only because he knows his mother is behind him.

In the course of the anal stage, the key personality in a child's life becomes the father—the one who gives his name to the child, who says "No," who draws the line and creates boundaries. The child feels able to blossom and develop within these boundaries, while without them he becomes unsure of who he is and how far he can go. This leads to hyperactive children who are always in to everything and push their mother to the brink. In situations such as these, we need to look at whether the father is present and whether he actually speaks to the child.

One evening in my clinic, I found myself face to face with an exhausted mother. Her child was extremely restless and wanting to touch everything—he'd run towards the remedy cabinet and his father would catch him just in time, then he'd run towards the scales and once again his father would grab him at the last minute. Finally, he started to go for my prized collection of Tintin figures!

Without moving, I let out a thundering "No!" The child stopped dead in his tracks, leaving the father flabbergasted. He realized at that moment that it wasn't enough to act out the "No," he needed to say it as well.


## CHILDREN WHO DON'T SPEAK

When the father is silent or absent, the child has difficulty finding its bearings and speaking its own truth, so that speech is significantly delayed. The remedy for this is often **Natrum muriaticum,** particularly if the child is thin, introverted, loves salt, and avoids the sun (symbol of the father in children's drawings).

Other remedies for delayed speech include:

**Agaricus,** where a disability means the child has physical problems speaking. Later, he will set out in search of the perfect words by writing poetry.

**Baryta carbonica** is intellectually slow, while **Nux moschata** prefers to sleep rather than confront the dangerous real world. **Belladonna,** meanwhile, is stuck in the oral stage and can't progress.

I often ask parents what they believe the father's role to be, and receive many different replies. The most common of these is that "He provides for the family and earns the money." I then explain that it is thanks to the father that we are able to leave the mother, and that without him we'd be at risk of losing ourselves in her. We need to progress from the infinite love of the mother to the no less infinite but carefully defined love of the father. The anal stage is therefore one of duality—of the choice between the father and the mother.


## IN THE NAME OF THE FATHER

The child's name and surname distinguish him from others and contribute to his personality. We find ourselves through others, because the only way we can discover who we are is by comparing ourselves to who we aren't. Otherwise, we'd all be the same, like in the Bible story of the Tower of Babel where at the beginning everyone had the same name and spoke the same language. Many a Fascist or Communist dictator has attempted to create a society of robots, of identical human clones who are totally incapable of original thought. We all know what eventually happens to such inhumane structures—the Towers of Babel always end up in ruins. Such was the fate of the odious system of Nazism and, several years later, of Stalinism—both of which were exposed for the criminal regimes they really were.

Some allopaths would like to see human practitioners replaced by computers, in order to ensure that the same prescription is given for the same complaint every time—regardless of patient, doctor, or country. This is yet another attempt to do away with original thought.

On the cellular level, lack of differentiation equals cancer—a disease that currently affects 30 percent of the Western population. These are people who have never really been able to say "No" and have allowed themselves to be invaded by beliefs which are not their own. Homeopathically speaking, this relates to Hahnemann's second miasm of Sycosis.

**Carcinosin** is the remedy for families with a heavy cancer taint, where every member will at some point develop cancer. These are very private people who avoid discussing important matters so as not to annoy others. They avoid all confrontation, conflict, and criticism and turn everything back onto themselves. They are actually afraid of the loss of love that such confrontation could bring, preferring to keep their ties with others at the expense of their own individuality.

Physically, Carcinosin patients are identifiable by the *café au lait* marks on their skin, their blue sclera, numerous moles and birthmarks, their sensitivity to music, and by their fussy, fastidious, and rigid personality, not to mention their extreme love of chocolate! Carcinosin children get none of the childhood illnesses, such as measles and whooping cough, but are especially prone to the "flu" (which will be helped by **Oscillococcinum**). They often have a lot of allergies and may undergo desensitization treatment—they long to be insensitive and immune to external stimuli, but forget that the purpose of life is to sense and experience.

**Ambra grisea** rejects the potty and hides behind pieces of furniture or waits for nighttime before going to the toilet. He is in fact stuck in the sadistic oral stage and runs away from smiling faces because he hasn't yet resolved his fear of being eaten. He believes that his excrement, and therefore a part of him, will be taken away and consumed. He is unable to see his stools as foreign substances and let go of them naturally. Later on, he is unable to rid himself of the negative things done or said to him by others and dwells on unpleasant matters.

This remedy is ideal for the social worker who spends all day listening to tragic stories and fails to protect herself psychologically, for the business man who lets himself be invaded by his customers, and for the doctor who can't cut the cords with his patients and wears himself out.

The key to Ambra grisea lies in our need to retain some level of detachment from the things that happen to us and to let go of all that is negative, ugly, and noxious without regret. In actual fact, we have nothing to lose and everything to gain. He who loses, wins.

Psychoanalysts have found one of the themes relating to the anal stage to be that of money, with the hoarding miser comparable to someone suffering from constipation. **Calcarea fluorica** is a good remedy for the miser, who can be identified not only from his avarices but also from his varices and varicose veins! His weak, loose-fitting teeth are prone to rapid decay since there is also a well-known connection between teeth and money, with children receiving a coin from the tooth fairy for every milk tooth they lose.

This connection between our physical selves and money continues throughout life. As people approach old age, they often attempt to replace the decaying material of their bodies with material possessions—a temptation which Confucius warned us against when he said: "In the third part of life, beware of the accumulation of material goods."

**Aurum metallicum** is for children who reject their father's authority. They are reckless daredevils who throw themselves into all sorts of dangerous situations. Later in life, they will seek to accumulate gold and money in order to become the father (God), bestowing their gifts on those around them—just as the sun bestows its rays. The only law they really want to follow is their own.

**Nitric acid** is obsessively rigid in his application of the law, with no mercy for those who break it. And yet forgiveness is essential to humanity if we want to put an end to worldly conflicts and wars. Mistakes are part of being human—that's why we make them. We only commit evil when we continue to make the same mistake after finding out that we're wrong. Jesus said we should forgive seven times seventy-seven times. Our reward comes in then being able to progress to a higher energetic level.

Those who know the Truth can no longer cheat and lie. The particular characteristic of **Veratrum album** is that he tries to lie his way out of everything, without realizing that this merely separates him more and more from reality.

The basic issue of Veratrum is his fear of losing his position in society. In children, this can manifest as a fear of losing the fusional bond with the mother when a second child is born. A typical scenario is that of the four-year-old girl whose development starts to regress during the mother's pregnancy. She becomes extremely bossy, vomits whenever anyone opposes her, and yet continues to suck her thumb or demand her bottle and pacifier. She is constantly inventing stories of princesses, and may even go so far as to tell the neighbor that her parents beat her.

We have seen how **Staphysagria** places itself in sadomasochistic or, most frequently, masochistic situations. His parents will describe their child as "always asking for a slap," because he seeks the evidence that he is loved and cared for in conflict, punishment, and humiliation. But in opposing others, we risk hurting them and being hurt in return—and so starts a vicious circle that risks ending in yet another case of child brutality.

The anal stage centers around the child's control of its sphincters and, by extension, its control of situations. It represents a progression to self-discipline and cleanliness and away from dirt, disorder, and anarchy.

**Sulphur** refuses to wash and loves being dirty. As a child, he will roll about in mud at the first opportunity. He doesn't want to learn anything and is so sure he already knows it all that he never listens to others. The anarchistic adult he becomes is easily spotted by the food stains on his shirt and the dirty fingernails.

**Aloe socotrina** refuses to gain control over his sphincters and stays in the oral stage. For him, to grow up means to eventually die—just like the aloe plant, which dies when its flower blooms and rises. These children don't want to learn to become civilized and they soil their pants (encopresis).

**Natrum carbonicum** is a hypersensitive soul who just wants to live in harmony. Unharmonious situations upset him and, like Aloe, he soils his pants. He can be identified by his gift for music, especially the piano. He has an aversion to honey, which his body can't tolerate even as a baby—if the mother's milk contains honey, he develops thrush. Made from sodium carbonate, this remedy balances states of excess acidity (i.e. of excess negativity).

**Medorrhinum** wants to control the passage of time, to know what will happen tomorrow, and he constantly worries about the future. Telltale physical symptoms include erythema across the buttocks, the frog-like sleeping position, onychophagy (nail biting), and astigmatism.

Finally, **Sepia** is like Cinderella—she cleans up carefully in the hope that this will get her noticed by the prince (her father). Sepia children sometimes have such a severe bout of chickenpox that they are left with a weak immunity and become prone to E-coli urinary infections (which may also indicate **Tuberculinum**).

We should mention here that chickenpox is typically an anal stage disease. The most frequently needed acute remedies are **Rhus tox** and **Mezereum,** especially in the itching phase. **Mercurius solubilis** will work wonders where there are spots in the mouth, while **Antimonium crudum** should be given if there's a concomitant cough.

The start of the phallic stage usually signifies the end of the anal stage. The child loses interest in its feces and turns all its attention to the genitals—its penis or clitoris. The child takes pleasure in exposing itself and running naked around the house after bath time, to the great amusement of its parents' friends! The main remedy for this stage is **Hyoscyamus,** and there is often an associated jealousy, such as that of the little boy who wants a penis as big as his daddy or older brother. Some exhibitionist adults are actually stuck in this stage of development.

This is also the stage in which little boys become inseparable from their sword or revolver, which they are constantly pointing at other people. **Ferrum metallicum** is especially fond of sword-fights and dreams of being a knight in shining armor.

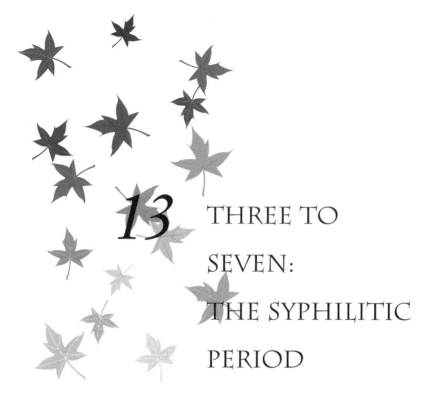

# 13 THREE TO SEVEN: THE SYPHILITIC PERIOD

It doesn't take too long before the child notices the special relationship between his mother and father—especially if this has tangible consequences, such as the birth of a little sister. Freud compared the child's jealousy at this stage with the Greek legend of Oedipus. When Oedipus is born, the Oracles predict that he will kill his father and marry his mother. The father therefore tries to get rid of the baby, but his efforts are in vain since the Oracles are proven right in the end.

So the first act of the Oedipal stage is the jealousy of the father who wants to kill his child. The psychologist Mary Balmary has shown how this can be compared with the Bible story in which Abraham drags his son Isaac out of his mother's arms and takes him into the mountains to sacrifice him to God, like a lamb. It is God who finally stops him and tells him to sacrifice a ram in the child's place. The death of the ram (father of the lamb) symbolizes the death of the father. Through this act, Isaac is freed from both his mother and his father and is able to establish his own identity.

Many fathers experience jealousy during the pregnancy, as their partner starts to build a fusional (and therefore exclusive) bond with the baby she's carrying. Some fathers never get over this experience—they feel unloved and go off with the first willing woman they meet. We are left with the fairly common scenario of the young single mother, abandoned by a man who couldn't or didn't know how to regain his rightful place in the family.

Some women have several children, each one by a different father who then disappeared during the pregnancy. In other cases, the father may push his partner into having an abortion, because he can't stand to have his position usurped by the new baby.

If the father does stay and manages to win back a place in his wife's bed and heart, the latter will gradually start to break the fusional bond with her child at around eighteen months. The child is very sensitive to this rupture and goes into a phase of extreme jealousy. He wakes up every night to go into his parents' bed, taking care to place himself between the two. He then sets about getting rid of the father, who is sick of losing sleep and having to go to work exhausted the next day. The father leaves his own room and spends the rest of the night in his child's bed. The child is then left to sleep alone with his mother—and so his Oedipus complex is satisfied.

In other cases, the child will make the most of family circumstances, such as the father going away on a business trip for several days, or holidays where everyone has to sleep in the same room. Some mothers indulge their children at these times, simply because fusional love is so fulfilling and so tempting.

The eventual rupture of the fusional bond can be so intolerable for the child that it goes into a deep depression. This can manifest as physical illnesses, usually affecting the left side of the body, such as left-sided otitis, left-sided mastoiditis, and left-sided lung problems. The child may even go so far as to endanger its own life, and in developing countries people talk of the child "going back." When I was working in Gabon, the families of my young patients often used to say to me, "Doctor, if the child wants to go, we should let him go."

In primitive societies, babies were suckled until they were eighteen months old and then abruptly replaced by their newborn siblings. Once "on the ground," they had to learn to eat manioc and plantains. Still in the anal stage, they would often choose a severe bout of diarrhea as the means to "go back," or else wait for the Oedipal stage and a left-sided mastoiditis.

The main homeopathic remedy for this state is **Lachesis muta**—the venom of the Bushmaster snake. Kent wrote that everybody needs a dose of this remedy at some point, since it enables us to get rid of the venom in our hearts. The human heart is like a serpent in terms of its character and desires—an image that is recognized the world over, since the heart is also one of the doorways to our collective unconscious.

The child needing Lachesis has murderous impulses—he wants to kill his father, but, since this is impossible, he takes out his violence and revenge on animals and other children. He bewilders his parents with his constant talking, which is his way of imposing his word—his personality. He has to be the center of attention all the time. Every time Mom is on the phone, for example, he starts being extremely naughty so that she will break the link with the other person.

The key to all this is actually the child's identification with the father. Little by little, he must stop his violence and learn to love others. But until then, he sees the husband as a parasite that needs to be killed. It is no coincidence that this is the time when children tend to have fleas, lice, and other skin parasites that need to be killed. Here again, **Lachesis** can prove very effective.

Cindy had started tearing out her own hair when her little brother was born and now had a large bald patch on her head. Lachesis quickly restored things to normal.

Stephen would go and sleep in his mother's bed whenever his father, who was a fireman, had to spend the night away from home. Every time his father returned, Stephen would fall ill—encouraged by the fact that his mother would then let him come back into her bed. This continued until the day Stephen's left tonsil started to hemorrhage badly and he had to be rushed into a hospital.

The father is said to be the ambassador of society, because it is through him that the child comes out of his Oedipus complex by renouncing exclusive, fusional love and moving towards an acceptance and love of everyone.

It is at this age that the teeth start to change. The milk teeth fall out and are replaced by new, permanent teeth. As we've already seen, the tooth fairy brings us a coin in place of each tooth—a part of us is taken away, and we receive in its place material goods.

However, we must avoid falling into the vicious circle of materialism, which later (and especially in old age) leads to the accumulation and hoarding of material possessions. The tooth fairy does not represent the accumulation of wealth, but instead the light-heartedness and love that should fill us whenever we lose something. Here again, homeopathy points to the truth—as a remedy is diluted and potentized, it progressively loses more and more on the physical plane and gains more and more on the energetic plane.

This ever-growing capacity to love others is the Third Dimension. We replace love of the "I" and of the "We" with love of all—of "One." It is at this stage that the child starts to ask existential questions—what happens to us when we die? What is there before and after life on Earth?

**Iodum** refuses to progress to this level and takes refuge in action, like Cain who was constantly working and finally killed his brother Abel out of jealousy. Abel was a shepherd who took time to think and contemplate, and Cain felt that God loved his brother more than him.

Iodum is an excellent remedy for the many cases of otitis media that occur around this time. The child hears everything through the liquid that has accumulated behind his eardrums, just as though he were still in the womb and surrounded by amniotic fluid.

Scarlatina is a childhood illness that is often related to the Oedipal phase. It is a disease that can provoke life-threatening inflammation of the heart and kidneys, with the main indicated remedies being **Aurum, Sulphur, Phosphorus,** and **Lachesis.**

**Cenchris contortrix** is for the morbidly curious child who secretly watches his parents and surprises them in the act of making love. He is deeply affected by the experience and turns jealous, naughty, quarrelsome, and violent, to the extent that he becomes a problem at school. As an adult, he will get a kick out of watching hardcore pornographic movies.

**Vipera berus,** the German viper, refuses to give in or lose anything because he fails to realize that life is about loss. He hoards everything, just like **Arsenicum album.**

**Castoreum** dreams of killing his father. It's a good remedy for phimosis and can enable the child to avoid surgery, which often leaves him with a deep fear of castration.

These murderous and destructive impulses relate to Hahnemann's third miasm of Syphilis—a disease in which the tissues are destroyed and anarchy rules.

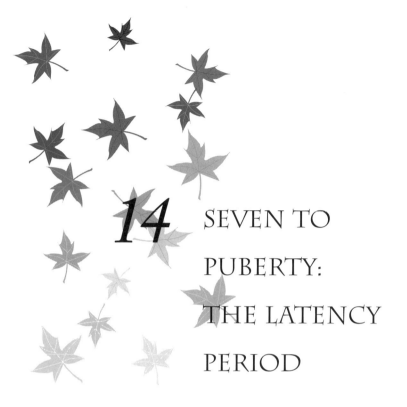

# 14 SEVEN TO PUBERTY: THE LATENCY PERIOD

Around the age of seven, the "age of reason," the child gives up trying to preserve the bond with the mother or to ostracize the father. Like Snow White, he leaves his castle to live with the dwarfs—the other children—and await puberty. All that's now left for him to do is correct his worst faults and acquire the intellectual knowledge offered him at junior school.

This phase of life brings few conflicts and consequently few illnesses.

**Taraxacum** is the pupil who does nothing unless there's someone behind him, urging him on all the while. It's getting going that he finds difficult. Left to his own devices, he would do nothing, or at most would spend all day playing with his friends, simply because he can't see any point in working hard. He has the characteristic physical symptom of a mapped tongue, which betrays an underlying liver problem.

**Calcarea phosphorica** is another good remedy for this phase of childhood. The Calc-phos child grows too fast and becomes thin, exhausted, and malnourished. School wears him out and he suffers from headaches because his intuitive brain is ill suited to the intellectual focus of learning. He is prone to swollen glands and can be so ticklish as to render any kind of physical examination impossible. He also has a characteristic voracious hunger at around 5:00 P.M. in the afternoon, just after school. Having devoured two or three sandwiches, he falls into an exhausted sleep and doesn't awake until the following morning. He can't bear any kind of injustice.

**Plumbum** can't stand rules and restrictions, especially those of school, which weigh heavily on him. His ideal would be to spend all day outdoors where he could observe nature, daydream, and play, and he just can't see the point of learning and copying. All he needs is a shot of lead—in homeopathic doses, of course!

Despite his bright and lively nature, the **Silica** child is so terrified before an audience that he retreats into his shell and avoids participating in class activities. Along with his constantly blocked nose and unhealthy, festering skin, he is instantly recognizable from his offensively sweaty feet.

**Baryta carbonica** understands everything, but too slowly. He feels ashamed because he can't keep up, and his classmates tease him mercilessly. His worst subject is mathematics, but a single dose of Baryta-carb will often enable him to catch up.

**Fluoric Acid** is too unstable to take in a whole day of lessons. His mind flits all over the place, imagining and daydreaming. Since he thinks faster than he can write, his workbooks are full of spelling mistakes. His key physical symptom is that his nails grow too fast and constantly need cutting.

## ENURESIS

Enuresis or bedwetting can hinder a child's social development if it discourages him from sleeping at friends' houses or from going on school trips.

The fact that animals use urine to mark their territory shows the usual source of the problem. There are many potentially useful homeopathic remedies, including:

**Kreosotum** and **Belladonna,** who sleep so deeply that they lose control of their bodily functions.

**Sepia** wets himself during the first part of sleep, while his days are spent tidying up in order to restore a sense of cleanliness and order.

**Capsicum** has never recovered from a house move or other displacement.

**Kali bichromicum** is trying to define his boundaries, just like an animal marking its territory.

**Lac caninum** is the main remedy for long-standing enuresis, which may continue through into adolescence. The patient believes he is worthless and that he will never achieve anything.

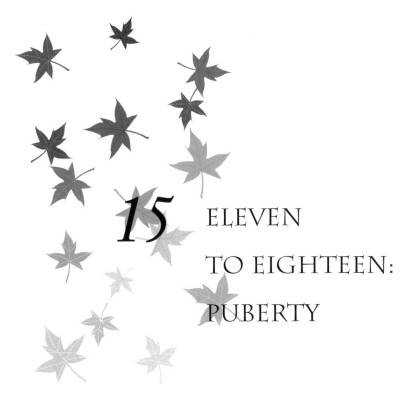

# 15 ELEVEN TO EIGHTEEN: PUBERTY

Formerly quite a brief phase in life, puberty has expanded out of all proportion in today's post-industrial world. Its underlying aim is to allow us to be born again, to pass into adulthood and discover who we really are—to "find ourselves."

## FINDING OURSELVES

**Cannabis indica** can't find himself, and if he breaks out of the family cocoon, it is only to enter another fusional relationship—that of the teenage gang where uniformity rules. They all wear the same clothes (sneakers, jeans, and T-shirt, preferably all in black—the color of the ego), and have the same thoughts and interests.

They will often share a joint of marijuana, in the unconscious search for the one remedy that would enable each of them to develop their individuality and so proceed on to the next phase— the girl-boy relationship. Unfortunately, it is only in homeopathic potency that Cannabis will prove effective. Material doses simply produce the opposite effect—disintegration of the personality with a fear of being drowned, as the teenager retreats emotionally to the waters and the fusional love of his mother's womb. He may eventually become psychotic, either from the cannabis itself or after moving on to harder drugs.

Cannabis has the effect of brutally separating the unconscious superego from the Shadow. The superego represents the limits and boundaries developed during the anal and Oedipal stages, while the Shadow is our instinctive, animal impulses. When the superego fails to control the deep impulses of the Shadow, there are no more limits. Car thefts, gang rape—literally anything goes.

Moving on to harder drugs is often the only way a person can see of integrating his spiritual dimension in a society that doesn't even acknowledge its existence. In Gabon, the illiterate Mitsogo people mark puberty with an initiation ceremony consisting of circumcision followed by the ritual drinking of *iboga* or "bitter wood"— a hallucinogenic substance that enables the youth to perceive the reality of soul and body through mystic experiences. It is after this rite of passage that the young adult is given his name or *koumbou*.

The drug dealers of modern society tempt the young with experiences of Paradise. But it is merely a fleeting imitation of Paradise, which is all too quickly replaced by the pains and torments of a hell that keeps them addicted. The dealers' work is rewarded with "dirty money"—a symbol of the anal stage from which they have themselves never progressed.

Entire countries have become willing accomplices to the drugs trade, since by providing anonymity and tax havens to its dealers they effectively launder the huge sums gained at the expense of our young people. The entire system needs to be controlled on a global scale, and as soon as possible.

As teenagers, each of us has to go through the developmental stages of childhood once again. The return of the oral stage brings with it the possibility of anorexia or bulimia. By not eating, the anorexic child attempts to deny the emergence of his or her sexuality, having not yet resolved the incestuous impulses of childhood. Anorexia is particularly common in girls, since losing weight often causes menstruation to be delayed or suppressed and prevents the breasts from developing. In this way, the girl stops being attractive to her father and can return to a state of fusional love with her mother.

**Tarentula** suffered early on from the excessive attention of his mother, who loved him too much and kept him tightly bound to her, as though in a spider's web. The child tries to escape by moving and dancing about frenetically, or by eating so little that he puts his own life in danger.

**Antimonium crudum** becomes bulimic in an attempt to forget her secret sorrow—the loss of the fusional bond with her mother. She is highly romantic and breaks down at each full moon.

The anal stage sees the return of certain obsessions, such as clothes and dressing up. The child becomes obsessed about his appearance, constantly checks himself in the mirror, and spends hours in the bathroom. These signs point to **Platina,** who confuses identity with appearance. Platinas give themselves away by two minor physical symptoms—their vision becomes blurred when looking at a bright light or a shiny object, and they get out of breath as soon as they start to run or walk fast (like **Digitalis**). Platinas are thoroughly taken in by the world of showbiz and celebrities and dream of becoming a star themselves some day. They get depressed in autumn, when the light (and the glitter) starts to fade. Then their only consolation is to spend a small fortune on themselves, on *haute couture* clothing. Platinas sometimes find their parents sadly lacking and may even believe they're adopted—they couldn't possibly have been born to such ordinary people!

Obsessive behavior also comes in the form of compulsive playing of video and computer games for hours on end, at the expense of books and schoolwork.

**Sulphur** never washes and takes to decorating the walls of his local town with obscene or scatological graffiti. The complete opposite of Platina, he only ever wears patched-up, dirty old jeans and sloppy shirts. His parents are "idiots" who don't understand anything, while society "stinks"—just like his teachers, who fail to appreciate his true genius. When he does take to reading, he chooses black, violent books where the reader is the hero and has to pass through hellish torments.

The syphilitic miasm and its destructive impulses cause some young people to join a revolutionary group, which may commit acts of violence. **Androctonus (Scorpion)** is the remedy for the morbid desire to break, kill, and destroy everything by violence. **Hepar sulphuricum,** meanwhile, is for those who want to set the world on fire in order to purify it and start afresh.

Fortunately, such impulses are usually played out only in the imagination. The teenager decorates his walls with morbid and obscene posters and, whenever possible, lets off steam by watching violent movies.

An unresolved Oedipus complex may lead the teenager to experiment with homosexuality. This is the young man who, having renounced the bond with his mother, sought in vain for love from his father and now hopes to remedy this lack with another man.

The "Don Juans" of our society indulge in uncontrolled sexuality, chasing every attractive woman in sight. They are addicted to falling in love, since this flatters their ego, but lose interest as soon as the woman gives in. They are constantly seeking fusion but never find it, since their only ideal woman was their mother!


## FORMING A COUPLE

Having fallen in love and formed a couple with the loved one, the teenager often expresses the internal conflict between the "I" and the "We" (the first and second dimensions of love) through a knee problem.

**Iodum** ruptures the cruciate ligament in his knee. Normally so active and industrious, with never a spare moment to stop and reflect, he suddenly finds himself nailed to the bed and forced to think.

**Medorrhinum** suffers from chronic knee problems. He sleeps on his stomach and sometimes even on his knees, in the Muslim position of prayer. He is in a constant state of anticipation so that, even at the start of a relationship, he often predicts how it will end and imagines the next one. He has multiple partners and runs the risk of contracting gonorrhea somewhere along the line.

**Antimonium crudum**'s love is unreciprocated, and he falls into a dreamy state of melancholy, especially around the time of the full moon, while during the daytime he releases his pent-up emotions by stuffing himself with food. The moon represents the fusional love of the mother, which Antimonium crudum misses so much. He seeks this same kind of fusion in his relationships and ends up scaring his partners away.

**Ignatia** wants to be with the loved one all the time. As we've already seen, it's the bean of St Ignatia who became literally ignited with love for God and wanted to be in communion with Him every day. The least separation produces sighing, listlessness, and physical symptoms such as a ball in the throat, as well as cramps, tics, and sore throats. Ignatias are introverted and never express their feelings but instead cut themselves off from others with their constant ruminating and self-analysis.

## SEXUAL INTERCOURSE

Most teenagers in Western societies have their first experience of sexual intercourse around the age of seventeen. The significance of this passage is different for girls than it is for boys, who don't usually commit themselves so much on the emotional level. In both cases, though, a large part of the teenager's vital energy becomes focused on sex and its twin poles of pleasure and reproduction.

The young adult has to deal with the risk of contracting sexually transmitted diseases such as AIDS while at the same time taking measures to avoid an unwanted pregnancy, all of which demands a certain level of psychological maturity. Those who don't take adequate protection may have to resort to abortion and the heavy emotional consequences that are involved in that decision.

**Conium maculatum** thinks of nothing but sex and his schoolwork starts to suffer. He needs to understand that energy goes to either the top of the body, to supply the intellect, or the bottom of the body, to supply the sexual organs, and that there's an appropriate time for each! His sexual frustration produces violent bouts of acne.

**Fluoric acid** goes from one sexual partner to another without any emotional commitment whatsoever. He wants the pleasures of physical love without the responsibilities it entails.

**Pulsatilla** is scared of men and avoids any situation that might lead to a sexual encounter. Paradoxically, her nights are filled with dreams of naked men.

**Cyclamen** withdraws into himself and spends hours listening to records in his half-darkened room, never going out, and dressing in black T-shirts with macabre designs on them. He would like to remain a pure spirit and avoids meeting people so that he never has to compromise. His education suffers and his marks start to go down.

## WORKING LIFE

The adolescent's choice of work will decide his or her future position in society. With competition for jobs and acceptance into colleges becoming more and more fierce, the young person needs to wake up and really go for it. This is possible if he feels that he's following his own truth.

**Anacardium** is unable to choose a career and finds it very difficult to commit himself to a single path.

**Baryta carbonica** is stuck in a state of embarrassed timidity that prevents him from taking any action whatsoever and slows down his mental faculties. He is especially poor at mathematics, with marks well below the pass rate.

As we've already seen, the difficult part for **Taraxacum** is getting going. He would be happy to spend all day playing cards with his friends in the local bar.

**Sulphur** can't see the point of making an effort, since he feels he knows everything already. He can be spotted from his sloppy, unwashed, and unshaven look and by his great philosophical speeches that are completely lacking in substance.

**Aethusa cynapium** almost immediately feels "stuffed" with knowledge and can't absorb anything else.

**Kali phosphoricum** wants to work alone, without any help, and becomes mentally exhausted.

**Gelsemium** can't stand examinations, which send him into a complete state of panic. He's spent the whole year studying but now can't remember a thing and becomes paralyzed with fear of making a mistake.

**Ignatia** spends too much time thinking about his emotional problems and lost loves to really commit himself to his studies. The day of the exam finds him in a state of panic, with lots of weeping and the sensation of a ball in the throat.

**Silica** is terrified at the thought of the oral exam, which means having to perform in front of others. And yet, once he starts, he does brilliantly. He sweats profusely from the hands and especially from the feet, making him an unpopular roommate. He also suffers from acne and unhealthy skin, with a tendency to suppuration.

**Kali bromatum** also suffers from acne. He doesn't want to study and prefers to earn money by stealing and cheating. His speech is faltering, and he may even stammer, while his nights are disturbed by nightmares.

**Carbo vegetabilis** can't make the grade. Extremely nervous in public, he comforts himself by smoking cigarettes that help to calm him down. His back is often covered in acne.

## LEAVING THE FAMILY

Eventually, each of us has to leave our family and move to another place—sometimes very far away.

**Pulsatilla** will do anything to avoid moving away from his mother.

**Bryonia**'s roots are too strong for him to envision living anywhere except the place he was born.

**Capsicum** is haunted by nostalgia for the lost paradise of his family home. He seeks comfort in overeating, which rapidly leads to obesity. He has a ruddy face and often drinks huge quantities of beer.

**Phosphoric acidum** starts to waste away after a move—he loses weight, feels drained of energy, and his hair (which is very greasy) starts to fall out. The drink Coca-Cola contains a lot of phosphoric acid, which helps to explain its popularity in the USA where most of the original population consisted of immigrants.

## PLEASURE AND SUFFERING

Teenagers find true pleasure in any act that enables them to "find themselves" a little, whether it be through lovemaking, a creative pursuit, sport, or some personal achievement. They want to push themselves to the limit, but first need to firmly establish their personality—their "I."

What the young person must understand is that in life we have two choices—either to have suffering first and pleasure after, or else pleasure first and suffering after. Drug addicts, for instance, choose the latter.

**Kali nitricum,** commonly known as saltpeter, is a highly explosive substance. It is the remedy for teenagers who wants to "break out" and have a good time, but whose ego is still too weak and fragile. A characteristic symptom of this remedy is eczema around the navel, showing an inability to come to terms with the cutting of the umbilical cord and separation from the mother.

Another explosive substance, nitroglycerine or **Glonoine,** is also a useful remedy for people who want to "break out" and who have the physical sensations of bursting and expanding. Their extreme intolerance of the sun is symbolic of their persistent intolerance of the father as a rival. People needing this remedy often suffer from explosive headaches.

**Baptisia** is a remedy for painless sore throats. It is good for young people who are attempting to assemble the scattered pieces of their own personality, like the pieces of a jigsaw puzzle. It is often needed by children whose families have been blown apart by, for instance, an acrimonious divorce.

## THE DANGERS OF SECTS

The re-emergence of the Oedipal phase during adolescence creates a desire for spirituality, which may tempt the young person to experiment with drugs. Religious sects represent another potentially dangerous alternative for teenagers seeking to fulfill their spiritual needs in a society bent almost exclusively on materialism. By offering ready-made answers, the so-called "guru" is able to channel all this youthful energy towards his own ego. Sexual energy and spiritual energy are one and the same, with the sole difference that one is focused in the lower part of the body and the other in the upper part.

Sects operate by isolating the individual and depersonalizing him so that he becomes homogenous with the group. The world outside is seen as diabolic, so that all contact with family and friends is broken off. When everyone comes to understand that spirituality is like a great mountain whose summit can be reached via many different paths, then, sectarianism will become a thing of the past.

**Bombyx processionea** (the Procession Moth) is the remedy for people who have effectively castrated their own personality in order to blindly follow "the Master." On the physical level, it is useful for twisted testicles—which can lead to actual castration. The caterpillar of the Procession Moth produces powerful allergens and is best left well alone!

**Spirituality is like a great mountain, whose summit can be reached via many different paths.**

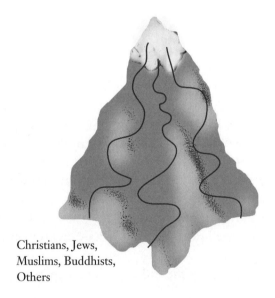

Christians, Jews, Muslims, Buddhists, Others

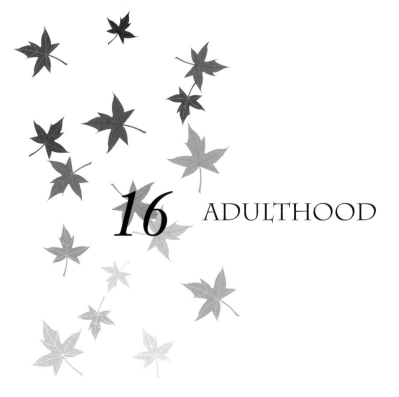

# 16 ADULTHOOD

After the white water rapids of adolescence, adulthood represents a passage into calmer waters. But there will still be opportunities to tackle any unresolved psychological problems, not least with the arrival of children.

It is as parents that we have to relive Freud's stages of development for a third time, and the fact that our children often closely resemble us makes this a fascinating experience. The first child's constitution often resembles that of the father, while the second child's is similar to that of the mother. Each parent comes face to face with his or her own qualities and failings!

Ideally, a mother should give her baby total, unconditional love throughout pregnancy and during the first few months, before allowing him to find his independence during the second year. At the same time, she has to manage the relationship with her partner and often her career as well. These three responsibilities don't always mix, and it can prove very difficult to be a good mother, a good wife, and a dedicated professional all at the same time—which helps to explain why so many couples break up. When this happens, there is an even greater temptation for the mother to withdraw into the relationship with her child. She may hold him in such a tight bond of love that he is later unable to cut the ties with the help of his father and thereby become autonomous. It is still tragically common for a child to lose contact with its father following a divorce.

**Sepia** presents the caricature of the woman who is permanently exhausted from having to manage not only the care and education of her children, but also the relationship with her partner and her professional life. Physically, she is chilly with ice-cold extremities, frequently constipated, and may carry a "mask of pregnancy" from her last child. Her weekend migraines enable her to dodge her "marital duties" and avoid falling pregnant again.

The father, meanwhile, needs to accept his partner's fusional bond with their baby during the pregnancy and avoid falling prey to extreme jealousy. Some fathers feel unloved at this time and become unfaithful, or they may even abandon the mother and child altogether in the search for pastures new. Sometimes the same scenario repeats itself again and again. Every time the woman becomes pregnant, she enters into such a total state of fusion with the baby that there is nothing left for the father and he leaves. Eventually, the woman is left with two or three children from different fathers, all of whom have vanished into the ether.

After the birth, the child's father needs to adopt the thankless role of boundary setter. He needs to be the one who says "No" and in particular, "No, you can't sleep in your mother's bed any longer"—thereby expressing this boundary verbally. Some strong-willed children react by turning their back on the father for several years.

Later on, the father—whose role is to introduce us into society—must be prepared to be overtaken by his children, to let them find their own way and do their own thing. This is especially true in adolescence, when the young person needs to follow his or her unique path rather than being a slave to his parents' views. This is what the Bible means when it says, "You will leave your mother and your father."

Finally, it is often the father who assumes the material responsibilities and worries of the family. The danger here is that his professional life will take over everything. Through fear of poverty, love of his work, or the desire for social recognition, some fathers become so caught up in their job that they end up being absent fathers. They too must learn to juggle their time, recognize that nobody is indispensable, and delegate to others.

**Nux vomica** is hyperactive and obsessive—everything has to be perfect. He over-extends himself with the abuse of coffee and other stimulants such as spices, pepper, and so on. Behind the façade, he has a fear of failure and poverty. His immediate problem is one of digestive overload, indicated by a yellow coating over the base of the tongue.

**Ambra grisea** wants to do everything himself and is incapable of delegating. Hopeless at setting boundaries, he allows himself to be invaded and abused and is extremely susceptible to other people's negativity.

**Lycopodium** overdoes it in his bid for power and bullies those around him, who have to be at his every beck and call. He only feels good when he's away from his family.

**Aurum** seeks social status. He needs to obtain gold, respect, and power so that he can then distribute his wealth to his entire extended family, but forgets to give the important things—time and love.

**Natrum muriaticum** is the father who never says a word. He always seems to be somewhere else, so completely absorbed is he by his own problems. He actually doesn't know how to communicate or talk about the little things in life, because he too had an absent father.

## DIVORCE

Children are always profoundly affected by a divorce, since they
are themselves the physical manifestation of their parents' union.
It is very difficult to have a successful divorce when the marriage
has been a failure! It takes great tolerance to see one's former partner settle down with someone else and be able to accept it. The
formation of new couples frequently leads to jealous scenes, which
are a throwback to unresolved Oedipal complexes. Children often
need **Ignatia** to help them come to terms with being separated
from one of the parents, and **Lachesis** on the arrival of their new
half-brothers and half-sisters.

Parents should take care to avoid criticizing the absent parent
in front of their children. A child is made half from the father and
half from the mother, so that half the child suffers when the mother
criticizes the father, and the other half suffers when the father criticizes the mother. The child ends up as a monument to suffering.

When a person divorces, he will often go back to being under
the thumb of his parents, who he has never left psychologically. I
saw one of my patients—a fifty-year-old father of three—move
back in with his seventy-year-old mother!

## ALCOHOLISM

It is because alcohol is such a good anxiolytic that adults often use
drink to forget their problems. However, they thereby run the risk
of becoming dependent and turning into alcoholics.

**Lachesis** is the typical drinker—lively and talkative but
extremely jealous, to the extent that he may turn violent. He seeks
fusional relationships and marries someone who will be as much
a mother to him as a wife.

**Nux vomica** gets angry at the slightest thing. He immediately
starts to swear and curse and may become violent, breaking things

and hitting out. Hyperactive and constantly overworked, he relies on stimulants to keep him going.

**Zincum metallicum** is for alcoholics who start to deteriorate on the neurological level. They have marked trembling and restlessness of the lower limbs, and often have an unresolved dispute with some authority figure or with the police—representative of their father, who was too strict with them when they were little and only ever expressed himself by shouting.

## CIGARETTE SMOKING

This is a habit that needs to be dropped before the whole family becomes ill through passive inhalation of tobacco smoke. Smokers are often people who have problems moving on to each successive stage in their lives and, as we have seen, use vegetable charcoal as a stimulant.

The children of smokers cough a lot, and the cause of many a Monday-morning cough is a preceding Sunday spent surrounded by cigarette smoke.

**Carbo vegetabilis** is the key remedy for helping people to wean themselves off cigarettes—something that should be done gradually, by smoking one less cigarette every day. **Tabacum** and **Caladium** can also be used as supports, if necessary. Caladium wants to live in a haze of smoke, so that he can't see the painful details of his life.

## TRANQUILLIZERS AND SLEEPING TABLETS

Tranquillizers are another trap to be avoided if at all possible, since they are highly addictive. So many people can no longer sleep or lead a normal life without the help of these "miracle pills," which enable them to avoid tackling the most basic issues in their lives. After several years of this type of symptomatic treatment, awareness, thinking, imagination, and memory all start to fail and the patient slides towards senility and loss of independence. They need to wake up, take the proverbial bull by the horns, and talk to someone who will really listen to them and accompany them on their internal journey. Every problem has a solution that we need to go out and look for—that is what it means to be a true adult.

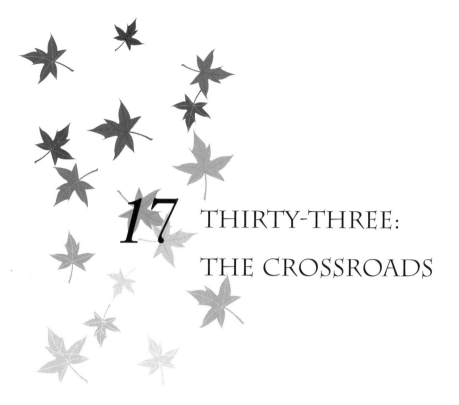

# 17 THIRTY-THREE: THE CROSSROADS

The passage from living as a couple to family life demands an ever greater amount of altruism, self-sacrifice, and self-questioning. The "We" gets bigger and bigger as the family grows, leading us towards the all-encompassing love of the "One."

Hindus believe it is around the age of thirty-three that incarnation of the *atman* (the personal soul or Self) takes place. It is the time when our soul, that eternal part of ourselves which existed long before our physical birth and will go on long after our physical death, comes into awareness.

The crisis is often triggered by something like a death in the family or an emotional problem, and may be somatized into the physical body as a frontal sinusitis (the place where Hindus locate the Third Eye—the eye of spirituality).

It doesn't matter which religion the person belongs to—it is as though a window opens, to reveal a new world which is more intense, more colorful, more vibrant. Nothing will ever be the same again, although the person's initial feverish agitation is gradually replaced by a certain degree of serenity. He devours one spiritual book after another—books about the hereafter, about symbolism, about life after death. He may feel the need to join a spiritual group, although here again he should beware of sects and their gurus, who like playing the role of the master and father (**Platina**) who must always be obeyed and whose beliefs take over our own. Jesus Christ told his disciples, "Don't call me master, you have but one master and he is inside you," and he bent down to wash their feet.

Some people refuse to give way to the spiritual dimension, which calls them towards reconciliation with others. They desperately hang on to the visible, material world, slam on the brakes of their spirituality, and demand proof. And proof is what they get—in the form of physical symptoms and in particular those affecting the liver, thyroid, and frontal sinuses.

**Arsenicum album** refuses to see beyond the material world and can't get over the death of a loved one. He becomes obsessive, miserly, and extremely chilly, and suffers from insomnia (at 3:00 A.M.) and frontal sinusitis. He wears black all the time, representing total ego and the absence of color and light. If his fear of death finally drives him to religion, he is likely to become the self-denying ascetic.

**Thuja** is the religious fanatic, consumed with passion for his faith. He wants to be in control of everything, to be at the center of the universe. He is the zealous disciple who may eventually become the master (like **Platina**).

**Conium** follows a succession of esoteric beliefs, each one more obscure and complicated than the last. He is a Gnostic who loses himself in intellectual theorizing and symbolism and misses the beauty in a rose or the spark in his neighbor's eye.

**Phosphorus** has indescribable, mystic experiences in which he leaves his physical body. He always seems a little "out of it," and may put his own life in danger through contracting pneumonia, hepatitis, or nephritis. He burns with all-consuming universal love and forgets that while still on Earth he needs to remain grounded. He has to work, earn a living, support his family, eat, sleep, and so on. Phosphorus would like to live on love and water alone!

Socrates said, "If a soul wishes to know itself, it needs to look at another soul."

So as individuals we can make much greater progress with someone else, starting with our partner. Couples hit a relationship crisis when the gap between their two personalities grows too wide. The remedy is simple—each partner needs to listen to the other and ask themselves what they could change in order to improve their relationship. Other people's criticisms always contain a grain of the truth that we've hidden away in our unconscious. We should never forget that our external relationships reflect our relationship with ourselves—between our conscious and unconscious selves. If something about our partner annoys us, it is usually because it reminds us of a part of ourselves that we refuse to confront or accept.

As we approach forty, we are faced with the most important choice in life—whether to favor matter or spirit. Depending on our decision, we become either materialistic or spiritual.

It is difficult to be materialistic without falling into a depression at some point or other, since matter is temporary—it can only deteriorate and always disappoints. Many depressives are people stuck in this cul-de-sac of materialism. They often have liver problems (problems with real living) and are "galled" by the fragility of material things. They don't understand that nothing on the physical plane really belongs to us.

**Chelidonium** is the remedy for liver pains in people who refuse to see clearly by opening up their Third Eye. If they happen to put some Chelidonium mother tincture on their warts, they will start to take great spiritual strides forward.

**Iodum** refuses to sit back and reflect and wears himself out with constant work. On the physical level, it's his thyroid that falls out of balance and becomes either hypo- or hyperactive.

Alain was suffering from progressive myasthenia and could no longer open his eyes, so that he seemed to be asleep all the time. Receiving an injection of iodine before a scan, he nearly died from anaphylactic shock. He was Jewish, and when I asked him what the word *iod* meant in Hebrew, he exclaimed that it was the first letter of God's name and burst out laughing. He explained, "I'm an atheist. So of *course* I nearly died when they injected me with God!" He was cured with a dose of Iodum in potency.

As for those who follow the spiritual path, they find themselves plunged into the third dimension of love. Altruism gradually replaces the ego, with its pride and its attachment to possessions and false certainties. Confucius said, "A man who has not changed before the age of forty will never change." Thanks to the discovery of psychoanalysis and homeopathy, this isn't necessarily true today. It does explain, however, why patients who are over forty often need to be approached from the material level, using potencies at the lower end of the scale (200C and below).

Elsewhere, Confucius wrote, "In the first part of life, beware of sexual excesses." The modern proliferation of sexually transmissible diseases proves him right.

A certain French film *(Ma Nuit Chez Maud)* shows how, through loyalty to his wife, the main character is able to spend a night discussing philosophy with a female friend without giving way to the temptation of having sex. At the end of the night, far from feeling frustrated, he feels strengthened by having been able to sublimate the huge amount of sexual energy released during their encounter.

When a baby is born, fidelity between the parents is a precondition if the man is to be able to identify himself as the true father and give the child his name. There are no such things as sexually transmissible diseases in the animal kingdom, but there is also no naming of the father and no access to the word. The word enables us to communicate fully using the upper part of the body and thereby progress on from the unbridled communication of sexual intercourse.

Confucius's next piece of advice was, "In the second part of life, beware of excessive striving." We need to avoid fanaticism of either the religious or material kind, remove our blinkers, and stay humble whatever the circumstances. If other people roll out the red carpet for us, we need to immediately ask ourselves where, when, how, and by whom we've been taken over. Each person holds the key to a part of the truth—nobody holds the key to it all. We need to love those who seek the truth, and be wary of those who claim to have the monopoly on it.

Finally, Confucius said, "In the third part of life, beware of accumulating material wealth." We need to do this by accessing the spiritual dimension and learning to share. True riches are to be found only in the spirit, which is the one thing that nobody can take from us.

These ancient sayings remind us again of Hahnemann's three miasms: Psora with its materialism and fear of poverty; Sycosis with its fanaticism and desire to control everything; and Syphilis with its unbridled sexuality. The world of advertising attempts to manipulate us through fear (Psora), money (Sycosis), and sex (Syphilis). So we have three different compasses, each of which points us in the wrong direction. Fear is a poor counselor, money can't make us happy, while unbridled sex destabilizes us by dispersing our energies horizontally and hindering our vertical progression towards spirituality.

It is around the age of forty that the individual, having now gained a certain maturity, feels ready to take on responsibilities other than those strictly relating to the family. He may signal this opening-up to the outside world by starting to play an active role in a union, society, or campaign group.

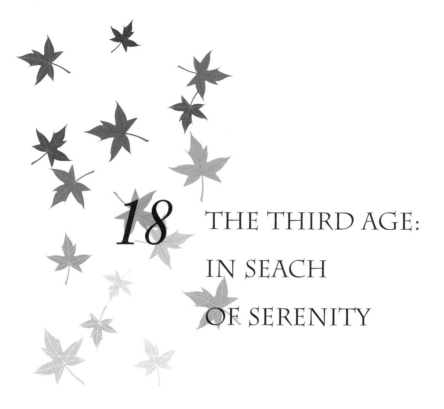

# *18* THE THIRD AGE: IN SEACH OF SERENITY

Hahnemann's three miasms make a fourth reappearance around the age of fifty. This is the time when children start to leave home and find partners and when grandchildren start to appear on the scene.

In women, the menopause heralds the end of physical creativity and the liberation of huge amounts of energy for spiritual creativity. Where there is imbalance, this energy may be channeled into other things—the woman may start to eat too much (Psora), become loud and controlling (Sycosis), or start destroying everything around them through jealousy (Syphilis).

Menopause is not a disease and women need to resist the temptation to start taking artificial hormones, as supposed "replacements." Hormones necessarily alter a person's psyche, and if there's one thing we need to hold on to more than anything else, it's our mind.

Loss of bone density after the menopause can be avoided with the help of homeopathic remedies such as **Calcarea phosphorica,** while circulatory problems can be relieved by the following:

**Lachesis,** with its ever-burning flame of jealousy, is the main remedy for menopausal hot flushes. It is useful for the woman who can't bear heat or tight clothing and who often wears purple. Her family and friends are worn out by her constant talking, which is exacerbated by her weakness for alcohol. She is constantly criticizing her son or daughter-in-law, or whoever she perceives as having stolen her child's love from her. She refuses to let her children go, failing to understand that—as Khalil Gibran says in *The Prophet,* "Our children are not our children. They are the sons and daughters of Life's longing for itself."

**Lycopodium** is the capable woman who tries to lord it over everyone. She suffers from abdominal bloating and bilious attacks and can't tolerate oysters, onions, and cabbage.

Covered in deeply cracked eczema, **Graphites** has stubborn constipation and is extremely chilly. She wanted to be a diamond, hard and clear, but remained dark and fragile. She needs to perceive her true role—as the pencil that draws the way.

**Kali bichromicum** is constantly "marking her own territory"—defining her boundaries with others, at the risk of making herself into the eternal scapegoat. She suffers from recurrent frontal sinusitis.

**Sulphuricum acidum** has hemorrhaging of dark, thin blood and hematomas all over the body. There may also be a desire or weakness for alcohol. People who need this remedy have never got over a physical trauma and live in constant fear of having another accident.

**Conium maculatum** is the stereotype of the elderly man who, instead of growing wise, becomes obsessed with sex. He has problems with his prostate, which is enlarged and may even become cancerous.

# FIBROIDS

These uterine growths may be so large as to make the woman appear pregnant. They usually symbolize a desire to conceive on the physical plane, at an age when we need to start conceiving on the spiritual plane. The womb also represents the household—the home, where children are made. This explains why women often experience a burglary as a sort of rape.

**Calcarea fluorica** develops a large, calcified fibroma. Her fear of poverty has driven her to accumulate material things, and this accumulation is reflected in her body.

**Phosphorus** can't progress to the third dimension in order to create on the spiritual level. She is constantly exhausted by her bleeding fibroids.

Those who *have* managed to resolve most of their issues by this time can now gain a new openness of spirit and a serenity based on knowledge and experience. They are able to transmit truth, beauty, and justice to others, and radiate the third dimension of altruistic love.

# FRACTURES OF THE FEMUR

The worst fear of the elderly, a fractured femur represents the inability to progress to this higher level of consciousness and a hanging-on to material things which then, literally, let us down.

**Arnica** is the first remedy to give in such cases. Made from an alpine flower that has spurred on many an exhausted mountaineer to the summit, the essence of this remedy is that it's all worth it. We are like donkeys, advancing through life with the help of both the carrot and the stick. In this case, it is the stick of our broken femur that drives us forward.

**Calcarea phosphoricum** can prevent fractures by restoring bone mineral content. A useful leading symptom of this remedy is hunger around 4-5:00 P.M., even in the elderly. These are people who dream of living in a fair world and who have a well-developed intuitive sense.

Once, when I was speaking at a conference in St Petersburg, an elderly Russian woman managed to push her way through all the barriers and get to the front of the stage, where she promptly demanded a consultation. My Russian colleagues tried to get rid of her, saying there was no time and that the program was full, but when I asked the woman what her problem was she said, "My bones keep breaking." I then asked her when she felt hungry. "In the afternoon," she said, so I prescribed Calcarea phosphorica 9C!

**Calcarea carbonica** is for those who have never managed to lose the fears we all have about our fragility as human beings. All through their lives, they have chosen safe situations and jobs— they are the typical civil servant. Often overweight, they would like to be as hard as rock, but remain crumbly and fragile like chalk.

**Symphytum** or knitbone is well known for its ability to promote healing of fractures. It's also the remedy for black eyes, bone pains, and pain in stumps following amputation (like Hypericum). Like Chelidonium, this plant can ease access to the third dimension.

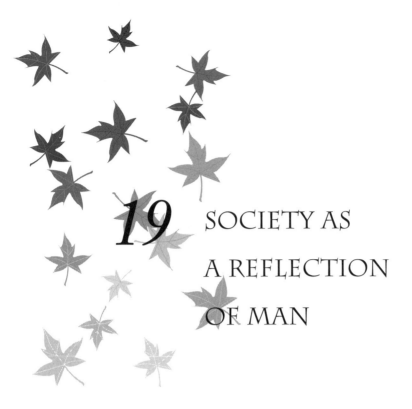

# 19 SOCIETY AS A REFLECTION OF MAN

Everything we've talked about concerning the evolution of man as an individual can also be applied to the evolution of human society as a whole.

As we've seen, a human being is like one vast community. It consists of billions of individual cells, each of which could survive on its own but which instead lives together with the others in a state of altruistic love. A heart cell beats for all the others, a foot cell walks for all the others, an intestinal cell digests for all the others. There are soldier cells to destroy intruders, police cells to direct the flow, and firefighter cells to put out any flames.

The ideal human society would therefore be based on the internal cellular society of a healthy human being. In the words of Hermes Trismegistus, "As above, so below."

Much of the world's population lives in undeveloped and developing countries, representative of the oral stage of development and Psora. People get up in the morning not knowing what they will eat that day or even *whether* they will eat. The search for food is the main preoccupation, and most diseases are due to poverty— leprosy, tuberculosis, diarrhea, malnutrition, even famine.

Another part of the world lives in a state of Sycosis, with all its attendant excesses—obsessiveness, acquisitiveness, money. It's the realm of stocks and shares, bureaucracy, and computerization. This is the home of the sadistic anal stage, with its tortures and cruelties that reached a climax during the last world war and remain only too common even today.

The results of such excess are cancer in all its forms, cardio-vascular diseases, and obesity. Cancer rates have increased in line with the risk from nuclear fallout, not least after the explosion of Chernobyl in 1986 when we all received a good dose of radioactive iodine. As we've seen, "iod" is the first letter of the Hebrew name for God. John's Book of Revelation predicted that "A great star fell from heaven, blazing like a torch, and it fell on a third of the rivers and on the fountains of water. The name of the star is Worm-wood (absinthe or Chernobyl in Ukrainian). A third of the waters became wormwood, and many men died of the water, because it was made bitter."

In a beautiful book entitled *De l'Homme-Cancer à l'Homme-Dieu* ("From Cancerous Man to Godlike Man"), Bernard Woeste-landt shows how only those who discover the third dimension are able to recover from cancer. In a sense, the cancerous cell has dis-covered physical immortality—it never stops growing and multi-plying, while normal cells die after just a few divisions. Cancer is a parasite that can only exist and develop by drawing on the reserves of the whole body. By wearing out its host, it only succeeds in exhausting and eventually destroying the organism upon which it depends. But a person who progresses to the third dimension effec-tively puts a limit on the cancer's development, says "No" to it, and receives a glimpse of true immortality—that of the spirit, in its compassion and love for others.

**The Miasmatic Cycle**

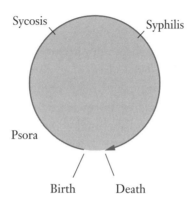

The Oedipal or Syphilitic stage concerns people who have a drug problem or issues around sexuality. They are particularly affected by the "modern" diseases—AIDS with its suicidal lymphocytes; hepatitis which reflects an inability to be a "liver" **(Phosphorus, Sepia, Lycopodium, Chelidonium);** and—latest addition to the many Alzheimers-like illnesses—Creutzfeldt-Jakob Disease.

## MODERN MAN

In developmental terms, Western society is nearing the end of adolescence. We are now faced with the challenge of progressing to spirituality and entering an adult, altruistic world in which all forces unite to create universal harmony and justice. The only alternative is to sink into the suicide of individual or collective madness.

In recent times, modern man has opened not one but two Pandora's boxes. The first was the opening of the atom, to reveal the enormous forces contained within. We now have nuclear energy and atomic bombs but still don't know whether we can control the invisible demons and avoid the threat that nuclear pollution poses to civilization.

The second opening was that of the cell nucleus, through genetic engineering. Once again, we are releasing forces we know nothing about. Will we be able to control them and avoid genetic mutations, which could endanger both the human race and the equilibrium of the plant and animal worlds? Already, entire nations are consuming genetically modified corn and soya and being inoculated with genetically developed vaccines (such as that for Hepatitis B).

We need to wake up from this state of semi-consciousness that materialism and its ego-centered temptations keep us in. We need to start saying "No"—asserting ourselves as individuals, rather than unquestioningly allowing our thoughts to be controlled by others. We need to maintain our creative individuality and reject uniformity. We need to share in order to remain young, forgive in order to stop hating. And most of all, we need to progress to universal, altruistic love and that state of bliss which makes the pleasures of the ego seem to fade into insignificance.

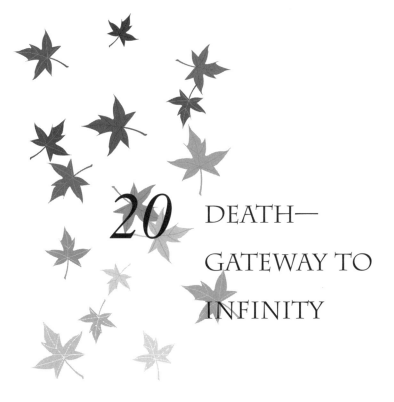

# 20 DEATH— GATEWAY TO INFINITY

Having run through the various phases of life, what can we now say about death? Death represents the beginning of yet another phase—the separation of the soul from the body and a final departure from material things and from Mother Earth.

In order to move on, our spirit must pass out through the head via the three meninges—the dura mater, representing the mother who didn't love us enough; the arachnoid, representing the mother who loved us too much and never gave us our independence; and the pia mater or "pious mother" who, having accessed the dimension of divine love, allows us to go our own way.

This passage is represented by the death of Jesus at Golgotha—the "place of the skull." At the last moment, he shouts in despair, "My God, why hast thou forsaken me?" So it is at this point that Psora, with its fear of abandonment, rears its head for the last time. Behind this final door, Love awaits us with the beauty of its light, knowledge, and truth. It is but a thin, opaque veil that hides this light from us during life.

Homeopathy can be very effective for those who are in the throes of death. It is at this time that we are often given a last chance to confront all our unresolved conflicts and put our house in order before the final departure. It is extremely important for the dying person to be conscious and surrounded by their loved ones, so that all can gain from the experience in terms of understanding and mutual love.

**Carbo vegetabilis** can't make the leap to the other side. He chokes, fights and refuses to go, all the time shouting, "Give me air, give me air. Fan me!"

**Arsenicum album** is terrified by the black wall of death, since he thinks there is nothing beyond. He clings to the physical world until the bitter end and thereby condemns himself to tremendous suffering.

**Tarentula cubensis,** remedy of the Cuban spider, can work miracles when nothing else seems to help the pain. The soul is held back by matter and the huge spider's web of Mother Earth. This remedy has the ability to rip open the web, thereby enabling the dying person to attain inner peace and leave his body. Thanks to this remedy, it is often possible to avoid using morphine until the very end and sometimes altogether, so that the dying person can remain conscious and make the most of his final moments on Earth.

# CONCLUSION

And so we come to the end of this superb journey that is human life on Earth.

We have seen how life is really nothing more than a love story. As Khalil Gibran says:

> *Love gives naught but itself and takes naught but from itself.*
> *Love possesses not nor would it be possessed;*
> *For love is sufficient unto love.*

Homeopathy is the ideal medicine to accompany us on our life's path. It is nature's way of providing man with everything he needs in order to be healthy, by helping him overcome each of the obstacles in his way. What's more, homeopathic remedies are practically cost-free and without side-effects, although Hahnemann emphasized the need for tireless enthusiasm and absence of prejudice on the part of the practitioner. My hope is that this book will have helped to fuel that enthusiasm!

I will end here with a quote from Sigmund Freud:

> *The intoxication produced by all out alcoholic drinks and stimulating drugs is but a pale reflection of that unique state of intoxication which is produced by love alone.*

# BIBLIOGRAPHY

Ancelin-Schützenberger, Anne. *Aïe, mes aïeux.* Paris: Desclée De Brouwer/La méridienne, 1993.

Aubier, Dominique. *Catalina ou la Bonaventure dite aux Français.* Paris: Le Courrier du livre, 1993.

Aubier, Dominique. *Deux secrets pour une Espagne.* Paris: Le Courrier du livre, 1982.

Balmary, Marie. *Le sacrifice interdit: Freud et la Bible.* Paris: Le livre de poche, 1995.

Chargé, A. *Traitement homéopathiques des maladies de la respiration.* Paris: LHF, 1977.

Cossé, Véronique. *Le coin du voile.* Paris: Gallimard, 1997.

Gibran, Khalil. *Le Prophète.* Paris: Casterman, 1987.

Hahnemann, Samuel. *Organon de l'art guérir.* New Delhi: B. Jain, translated by W. Boericke, 1921.

Lecarrière, Jacques. *La poussière du monde.* Paris: Nil Editions, 1997.

Salomé, Jacques. *T'es toi quand tu parles.* Paris: Albin Michel, 1991.

Schuré, Edouard. *Les grands initiés.* Paris: Le livre de poche, 1983.

de Souzenelle, Annick. *De l'arbre de vie au schéma corporel.* Paris: Albin Michel, 1991.

de Souzenelle, Annick. *La symbolique du corps humain.* Paris: Albin Michel, 1991.

de Souzenelle, Annick and Jean Mouttapa. *La parole au coeur du corps,* Paris: Albin Michel, 1997.

Tisseron, Serge. *Tintin et les secrets de famille.* Paris: Seguier, 1990.

Woestelandt, Bernard. *De l'homme-cancer à l'homme-Dieu.* Paris: Dervy, 1995.

# INDEX

# Related Homeopathy Titles from
# North Atlantic Books

**Discovering Homeopathy:**
**Your Introduction to the Science and Art**
**of Homeopathic Medicine**
By Dana Ullman
ISBN: 1-55643-108-2
$16.95 trade paper, 312 pp.
With a foreword by the Physician to the Queen of England, Ullman's book provides an overview of the homeopathic approach to understanding and treating common ailments. Ullman includes sections on homeopathy's history, a modern understanding of homeopathic medicine, specific issues from women's health to sports medicine to pediatrics, and homeopathic resources.

**The Homeopathic Emergency Guide:**
**A Quick Reference Handbook**
**to Effective Homeopathic Care**
By Thomas Kruzel
ISBN: 1-55643-123-6
$22.95 trade paper, 384 pp.
Dr. Thomas Kruzel's *Homeopathic Emergency Guide* is a handbook to assist the practitioners of homeopathy with the task of individualizing cases. Since the book is organized by diseases and symptoms, the case taker can compare the totality of symptoms with remedies and more easily select the right remedy.

**Homeopathic Medicines for Pregnancy and Childbirth**
By Richard Moskowitz
ISBN: 1-55643-137-6
$16.95 trade paper, 312 pp.
This book offers an introduction to the philosophy and practice of homeopathy, as well as case presentations for mother and child, including labor pain, teething, depression, irritability, and marital discord.

**Homeopathic Psychology:**
**Personality Profiles**
**of the Major Constitutional Types**
By Philip Bailey
ISBN: 1-55643-099-X
$25.00 trade paper, 440 pp.
The thirty-five most common personality types recognized by homeopathic practitioners are brought to life by Bailey. The types are described in light of common behaviors, primary emotional tendencies, internal conflicts, and spiritual issues that each of them face.

**The Homeopathic Treatment of Children:**
**Pediatric Constitutional Types**
By Paul Herscu
ISBN: 1-55643-090-6
$22.50 trade paper, 390 pp.
"This is a reference guide for parent and doctor alike. It is hoped that by reading this book you will better be able to report recognizable symptoms and personality traits to your homeopath, so that he or she in conjunction with you will be better able to find the remedy that will help your child."
—from the book

**Homeopathy: The Great Riddle**
By Richard Grossinger
ISBN: 1-55643-290-9
$14.95 trade paper, 192 pp.
A thorough explanation of homeopathy for the general reader, *Homeopathy: The Great Riddle* addresses the mystery of how a medicine using spiritual doses can cure deep-seated physical diseases.

"Grossinger's lucid, informative, and sympathetic account demonstrates how homeopathic theory is itself a critique of standard medical practice."
—*Publishers Weekly*

**Homeopathy: Science or Myth?**
By Bill Gray
ISBN: 1-55643-332-8
$14.95 trade paper
216 pp., illustrations
"Dr. Gray has competently spelled out in easily understandable terms the scientific foundation underlying homeopathy."
—George Vithoulkas, recipient of the "Alternative Nobel Prize for Health," 1996

"Both clinicians and patients can look forward to this volume playing a significant role in the evaluation and acceptance of homeopathy into the exploding field of integrative medicine."
—Kenneth Pelletier, Director of the Complementary and Alternative Medicine Program at Stanford University (CAMPS)

**Homeopathy for Musculoskeletal Healing**
By Asa Hershoff
ISBN: 1-55643-237-2
$20.00 trade paper
328 pp., illustrations
Musculoskeletal problems—including low back pain, migraine, a sore neck—are the most pervasive and debilitating conditions in our culture, causing untold pain. This book contains practical information for both consumers and clinicians and various helpful charts and diagrams for prescribing cures.

**Psyche and Substance:**
**Essays on Homeopathy in the Light of Jungian Psychology**
By Edward Whitmont
ISBN: 1-55643-106-6
$16.95 trade paper, 256 pp.
Whitmont explores the archetypal and morphological dimension of homeopathy through his essays and case studies.

"Above all else, Whitmont's life-affirming philosophy places these archetypal patterns in a historic context extending from medieval alchemists to molecular biologists and restores a sense of balance to the dynamic which is life itself."
—Kenneth Pelletier

**The Spirit of Homeopathic Medicines:**
**Essential Insights to 300 Remedies**
By Didier Grandgeorge
ISBN: 1-55643-261-5
$20.00 trade paper, 240 pp.
Grandgeorge traces the common thread connecting our physical suffering and unconscious motivations. He matches more than three hundred homeopathic remedies to the emotional substructure underlying physical ailments.

**Sports and Exercise Injuries:**
**Conventional, Homeopathic, and Alternative Treatments**
By Steven Subotnick
ISBN: 1-55643-114-7
$18.95 trade paper
432 pp., illustrations
From rheumatoid arthritis to heel spurs, Dr. Subotnick's book guides readers through the healing process from sports and exercise injuries via a range of remedies, including sports massage, bodywork, movement, and psychotherapy to homeopathy and internal martial arts.